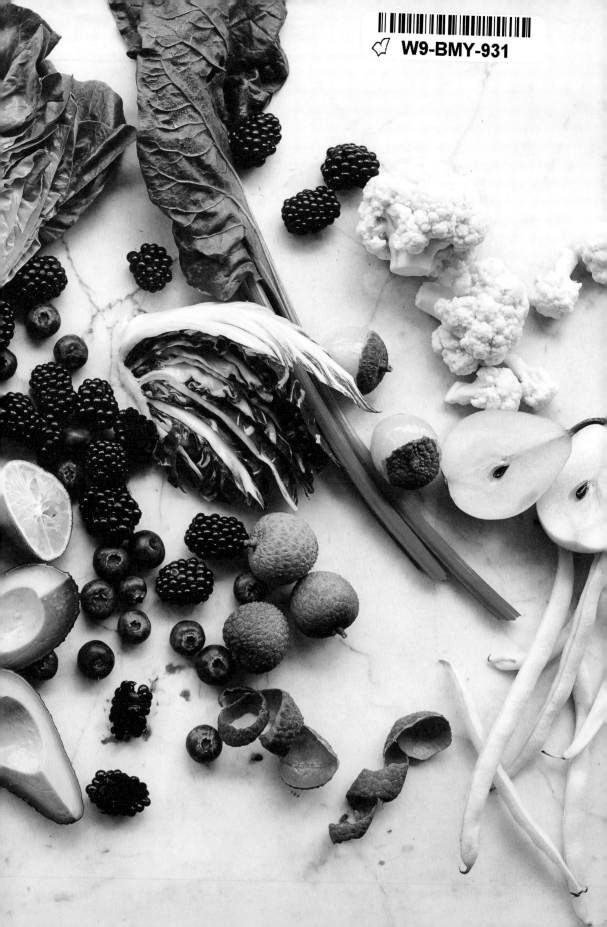

THE
Yoga Kitchen
PLAN

A SEVEN-DAY VEGETARIAN LIFESTYLE PLAN
WITH OVER 70 RECIPES

KIMBERLY PARSONS

Photography by Laura Edwards

Hardie Grant

QUADRILLE

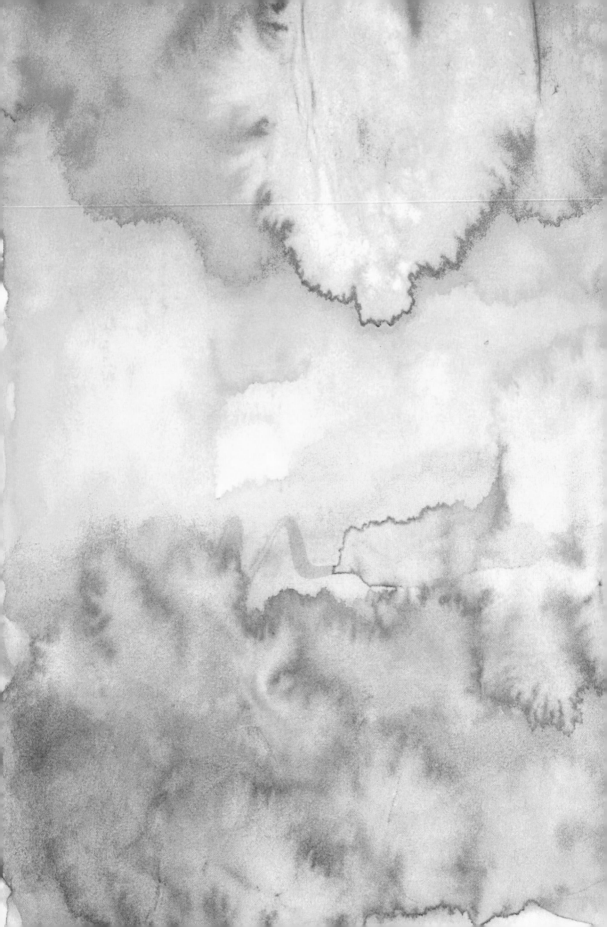

CONTENTS

WELCOME TO THE
YOGA KITCHEN PLAN

Welcome to *The Yoga Kitchen Plan* and way of life!
This is your seven-day yoga lifestyle and four-week
vegetarian meal plan which will take you on a personal
and spiritual journey as you transition through the
chakras each day.

You will cultivate daily yogic habits through the seven-
day lifestyle regime to further your inner yoga practice
and live the yogi's way of life. You will also nourish
your mind, body and soul with your choice of three
easy-to-prepare daily meals using my healthy-eating
principles for optimal calm, clarity and energy.

You will delve deeper into a traditional way of yogic
eating, following a sattvic (pure) food model. The food
is lacto-vegetarian, meaning fruit, vegetables and dairy
predominate in the diet, while you exclude stimulating
foods, such as eggs, garlic and onion and foods
containing caffeine, because these unsettle the mind.

It is my hope that this book will bring you closer
to an authentic inner connection with yourself and
complement your yoga journey to help you find true
inner peace and freedom.

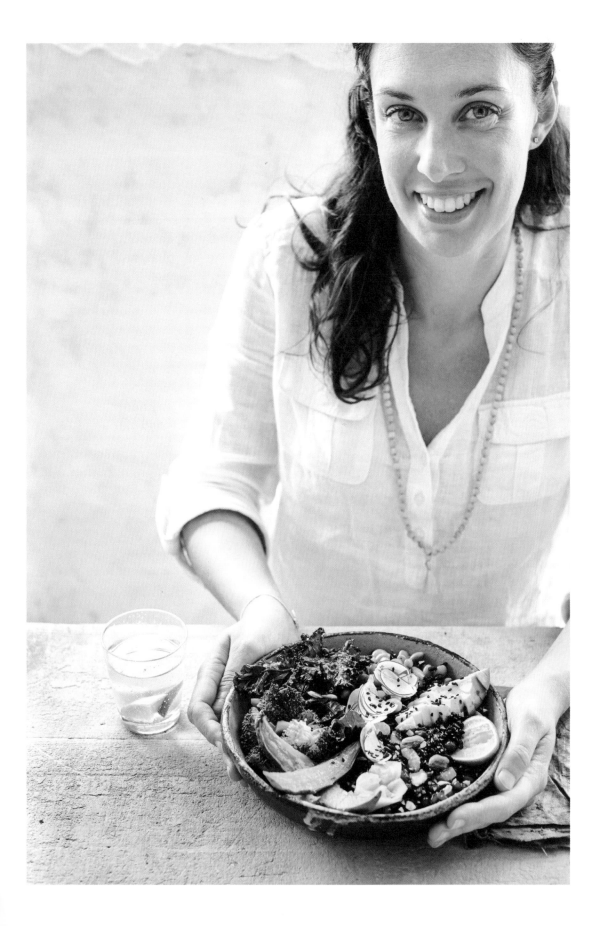

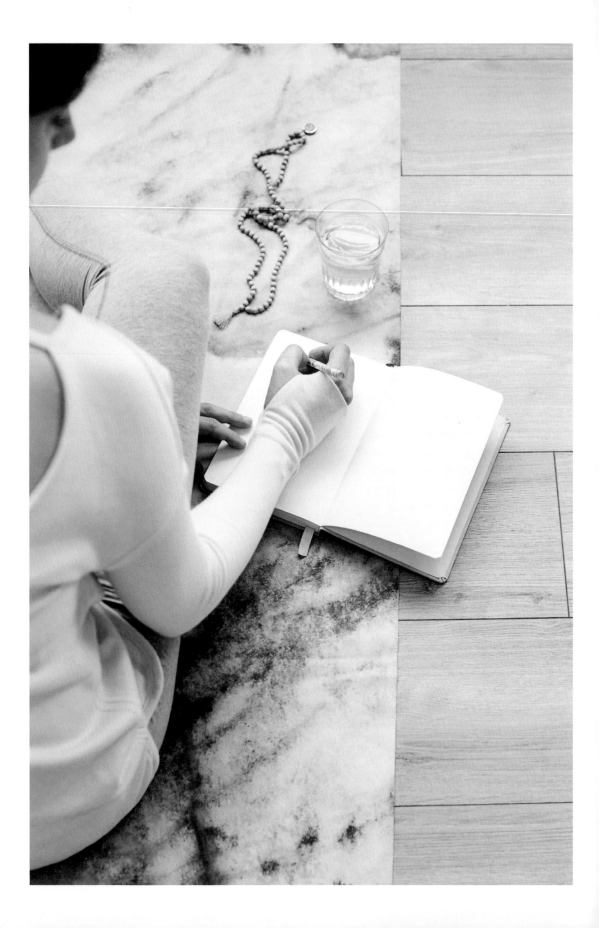

WHY THE YOGI WAY OF LIFE?

What I have come to realize about yoga through my own practice is that living a yogi's life is the real yoga challenge. All the effort I pour into my asana practice on the mat is just a testing ground for the way I act and how I apply these yogi values in my life. I have come to accept yoga as a physical discipline with a spiritual intention, because the art of being kind all day, speaking only truthful statements and remaining calm when faced with difficulty can sometimes feel impossible. But these objectives are worth the challenge in more ways than one.

From a physical point of view, yoga lowers stress and improves posture, circulation and digestion while keeping joints fluid and muscles toned. It can help you lose weight and alleviate symptoms of depression, and it may also be the best anti-aging regimen we have. Yoga also eases everyday pains and frustrations and increases kindness and compassion. It tones the body while stabilizing the mind.

In the ancient language of Sanskrit, the word *yoga* is used to signify any form of connection. When applied to the human experience, it can be used to celebrate the union between the mind, body and spirit. At its most practical level, yoga is a process of becoming more aware of who we really are. Through its practices, we can still the mind and merge into oneness with the divine, to act with truth and authenticity.

Over the years I have had the privilege of witnessing first-hand the positive changes that the daily combination of asana practice and healthy eating can achieve in our lives. The guests on my many yoga retreats have been my teachers and shown me just how powerful this combination really is when put into practice. It is my mission through *The Yoga Kitchen Plan* to help as many of you realize this powerful union and reach the same state of blissful calm, clarity and wellness that my guests achieve while on retreat.

THE CHAKRA ENERGY SYSTEM

The seven-day lifestyle plan is based on the chakras – the wheels of energy throughout the body. There are seven main chakras, starting from the base of the spine through to the crown of the head. To visualize a chakra in the body, imagine a swirling wheel of energy where matter and consciousness meet, with the wheels perfectly aligning up and down the spinal column. I often help others to visualize the energy pulsing through their body by using the lymphatic system as a physiological comparison. The lymphatic system covers every part of the human body with vessels that sit just under the skin's surface. Imagine energy pulsing through these vessels, travelling to the chakra 'wheels', which you can imagine as the lymph organs or nodes. The chakra 'wheel' for each of the seven chakras is where the energy for that particular chakra accumulates and is processed just as our lymph fluid is within the lymphatic system.

The invisible energy pulsing through this system is vital life force, chi or prana, which keeps us vibrant, healthy and alive. Each of the seven chakras has an important part to play in our overall energetic balance and has long been the traditional method for yogis to understand the anatomy of the subtle body. To translate and help us better understand the practical benefits of the chakras, I have outlined three main areas here:

ACHIEVE BALANCE

By focusing your attention on one or more characteristics of each chakra, you can subtly encourage the qualities it stands for into your life. By devoting your awareness to the subtle energy of each chakra, such as security, power, love or insight, you can activate this potential.

DEVELOP ENERGETIC FLOW

Traditionally, chakras are the known 'gateways' through which our life force, chi or prana energy is able to move through our mind and body. This energy gets transformed into mental, physical and emotional expressions such as 'support', which is a key characteristic of the root chakra, and is associated with feelings of independence, belonging and stability.

A practical approach towards feeling in 'flow' with your energies is to examine your relative strength or weakness for the individual chakra characteristics, so you can improve where you feel weak (physically, mentally or emotionally) and expand where you feel strong.

ENHANCE WELLBEING

The chakras allow us to organize our life and body into an all-inclusive and whole being. From this space we can gain access to the subtle levels of life where hidden potentials can be activated and greater fulfilment is born.

During the plan I have created, you will move from chakra to chakra each day, starting at the root chakra where you will focus on finding your earth and a stable base, i.e. who you are at your essence. Then, over the seven days, you will ascend to the crown chakra where true connection with your consciousness awaits you.

THE INDIVIDUAL CHAKRAS

As well as its individual characteristics, each chakra is associated
with a colour. See pages 16 to 29 for more information.

ROOT CHAKRA
Survival / Grounding / Stability
Security / Safety / Support / Family
A Sense of Belonging / Community

When you need to feel safe, secure,
passionate, energetic, balanced,
vibrant; for a sense of belonging and
community; to create a sanctuary for
you to feel 'home'.

SACRAL CHAKRA
Relationships / Sexuality / Empathy
Pleasure / Wellbeing / Connection
Change / Feelings and Emotions
Creativity

When you need to feel confident,
connected to everything around you
and yourself; to deal with change
and develop relationships with others;
to help you move your body, feel
pleasure, express your sexuality.

SOLAR PLEXUS CHAKRA
Will / Power / Joy / Motivation
Self-esteem / Transformation
Identity / Vitality

When you need to feel energized,
determined, powerful, happy, joyous,
hopeful; when you need a sense of
empowerment or standing steady
in your own self; to express your
individuality and provide willpower.

HEART CHAKRA
Compassion / Love / Open-
heartedness / Desire for Self-
acceptance / Balanced
Emotions / Harmony / Forgiveness
Gratitude / Devotion / Nurture / Heal

When you need to feel nourished,
loved, natural, youthful, rejuvenated,
intelligent; when you need to cultivate
gratitude and healing in your life.

THROAT CHAKRA
Communication / Self-expression
Truth / Authenticity / Integration

When you need to speak and hear
the truth and live authentically; to feel
tranquil, steady and integrated in your
internal and external worlds; when
your heart and mind are in conflict.

THIRD-EYE CHAKRA
Knowingness / Intuition / Perception
Wisdom / Imagination / Meditation
Self-reflection

When you need to concentrate and
focus; to cultivate sophistication,
mystery and wisdom; to boost your
perspective and imagination.

CROWN CHAKRA
Consciousness / Unification / Purity
Bliss / Divinity / Spirituality
Simplicity / Clarity

When you need to feel cleansed,
pure, clear; when a sense of spirit
and connectedness abound; where
intentions live alongside the connection
to your higher consciousness.

PRANAYAMA

Let's explore the very foundation of all yoga: the breath. Although you may often take it for granted, your breath not only keeps you alive by oxygenating your body, but also keeps you connected to your energy within. Breath is the link from your soul to your body, your mind and your emotions. It nourishes you and is always there for you. It is like sending an email to your nervous system with the simple message to relax.

During yoga, you are often instructed to inhale and exhale; it is through this conscious breath work that you are able to navigate the different levels of your consciousness. Connecting to your breath grounds you in the present moment, allowing you to let go of the past and future and focus solely on the moment inside the breath. This is why conscious breathing can be its own form of meditation. Cultivating a conscious breathing practice will become one of your daily yoga habits in *The Yoga Kitchen Plan* and I am going to show you how easy it is to include in your daily life. But first let's step a little further into why conscious breath is so good for you.

Often, your mind is thinking about something while your body is doing something else. As a result, your mind and your body are not unified. Becoming aware of your inhalation and exhalation, you bring your mind and body to work together because both are focused on the same thing and when you breathe consciously you activate a different part of your brain. Unconscious breathing is controlled by the medulla oblongata in the brain stem, the primitive part of the brain, while conscious breathing comes from the more evolved areas of the brain in the cerebral cortex. By activating the cerebral cortex when you breathe deep into your belly, you give the indication to your mind that you are relaxed. On a physical level, deep belly breathing also brings more oxygen to all of our body.

In essence, by consciously breathing, you are controlling which aspects of your mind dominate, therefore causing your consciousness to rise from the primitive and instinctual to the evolved and elevated – the perfect state for yoga! However, the true magic of breathing starts when you master the exhalation of your breath. During inhalation, the mind is calmer and one can hold the breath longer without experiencing any form of discomfort. But after exhalation there is a natural urge to inhale immediately. When this natural tendency calms down, you will be able to reach a higher level of consciousness. Luckily for you, I have the perfect breathing technique to help you master the art of calming your mind between the exhalation and inhalation of your next breath.

By breathing, you also rid your body of waste products and toxins. However, most of us use only one third of our actual breathing capacity and so our cells are not able to eliminate the toxins from our bodies as easily.

Outlined below are the three conscious breathing techniques you will use as part of the daily yoga lifestyle plan. If at any time you need to remind yourself of the techniques, simply flick back.

*Note for pregnant women – Focus on developing awareness of your breathing, rather than holding your breath. Yoga experts recommend pregnant women should avoid holding the breath for any period of time. Also avoid taking deep, quick, forceful breaths, as this can lead to feeling faint, light-headed and dizzy.

BREATHING EXERCISES

THE BREATH OF LIFE

In the morning, deep breathing awakens your senses by oxygenating every cell in your body and helps your body dispel sleep-induced toxins.

1. Stand with your arms by your sides. Exhale through your nose, emptying your lungs completely (ideally, all inhales and exhales should be through your nose).
2. Immediately inhale deeply through your nose, slowly bringing your arms up over your head and bring your palms to touch, then pull up on your toes, raising your heels as far off the ground as possible.
3. Hold the breath for the count of five.
4. Now slowly exhale fully through your nose until all the breath has been released, slowly lowering your arms to your sides and replacing your heels on the ground.
5. Hold the breath for the count of five.
6. Repeat the exercise ten times, without pause.

The exercise can also be performed from a sitting or lying position. Omit the arm movements if you're lying down on your back.

1. Breathe evenly, focusing on the movement of your stomach. Let your stomach rise up to bring air into the lower part of your lungs. As your lungs fill with air, your chest begins to rise while lowering your stomach. During this time, you must not strive. The length of the exhalation will be longer than the inhalation.
2. Repeat the exercise ten times, without pause.

A WALKING MEDITATION

This is a walking meditation with a breathing exercise as the main component. It will become part of your daily routine and is best done to the beat of your steps while walking. It doesn't need to be a long walk – try three to five minutes as you walk to work. It's the perfect way to find calm amid the chaos of the day and remind you of the inner strength and peace you cultivate in your morning meditation.

1. As you start to walk, become aware of the regular pace of your steps. Start by counting 20 paces and bring attention to how each foot goes back down to earth with every step. Notice how the outer parts of your feet touch the ground and how your toes feel as they find the ground. Bring all your attention to your feet and these first 20 paces.
2. Now take a deep breath in and count to four while taking four steps.
3. Then hold your breath for the next four steps.
4. Then exhale for the next four steps.
5. Then hold again for the next four steps.
6. Repeat the inhale to the count of four steps. In your mind you can say to yourself 'inhale two, three, four; hold two, three, four; exhale two, three, four; hold two, three, four'.
7. Focusing on the breath and the count of four, repeat the process until you become relaxed.

WALKING INTO GRATITUDE

If you'd like to bring some gratitude into your walking meditation, try this technique.

1. Inhale and begin your count of two, three, four. Think of someone you're thankful for in your life (quick: you've only got four counts).
2. Hold and count two, three, four and think of something from today that you're thankful for.
3. Exhale and count two, three, four and think of something from nature you're thankful for.
4. Hold and count two, three, four and think of something else from today you're thankful for.
5. Continue this pattern for as long as you can continue to think of things to be grateful for.

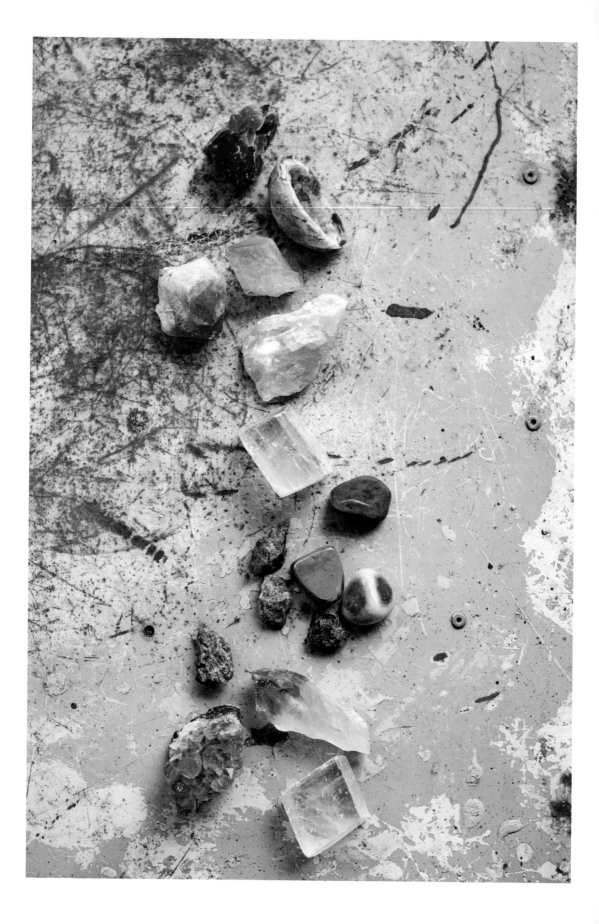

THE YOGA KITCHEN
SEVEN-DAY LIFESTYLE PLAN

Most people associate yoga with an asana practice, but yoga isn't just about flowing through a series of poses, twisting yourself up like a pretzel and sweating your butt off (though that part is fun and highly beneficial both physically and mentally). Yoga is also about how you live your life in all contexts.

While the yoga poses are certainly a key aspect of the tradition, they are just one part of a much bigger picture. Written over 2,000 years ago and considered the foundation of classical yoga philosophy, values and principles, the *Yoga Sutras* laid out by Patanjali outline our inner yoga journey. They are filled with a wealth of knowledge to light a path towards a steady, calm and peaceful mind.

With Patanjali's sutras in mind, I have created your very own daily yoga lifestyle plan, bringing to life the fundamental values and principles of these sutras in real and tangible daily techniques. This plan aims to awaken you to your spiritual path, giving you a daily yogi practice that's separate from your asana practice. This is the real yoga; the truest test of your discipline towards reaching freedom and peace in your mind. Follow these daily lifestyle practices to transform into a happier, healthier, more vibrant, stress-free you.

HOW TO FOLLOW THE PLAN
Choose any day in the week, and begin! If you miss a day, don't worry; just restart the following day. We are human and our yoga transformation has no room for perfectionism, so if you follow only part of the plan each day then pat yourself on the back and look forward to the next day. Enjoy this voyage towards your inner yogi.

THE DAILY TECHNIQUES
WAKING WITH THE SUNRISE
In order to fit in a fantastic morning, you're going to need some extra time compared to your normal routine. So if you favour the peace and quiet a late night affords, you'll be equally satisfied by the same peace and quiet an early morning provides, and it's simply a matter of shifting your personal time to the morning rather than late at night. Waking with the sunrise also helps you to connect to the natural rhythm of the Earth we live on and universe we exist within.

BODY SCAN
Listening to your body and acknowledging the signs and symptoms it may be giving you is an integral part of learning how to look after your body and knowing what it needs. Body scanning is easy and should only take 30–60 seconds to complete.

Upon waking, in that moment just before your brain engages in the day's activities, allow yourself to have a moment with your body to scan for any signs or symptoms it may be indicating to you. These may include a dry mouth, bloating, aches or pains, stiffness of muscles or joints, hunger, thirst, sexual arousal or a headache.

Keep a notepad next to your bed and jot down the top three things you notice each morning. Over the course of the week, patterns may emerge. Each day I will ask you to focus your attention on a different part of your body, which will help you assess each chakra.

ASANA PRACTICE
After your body scan, empty your bladder and bowels as required and put on some comfortable clothes for your asana practice.

13

Roll out your mat and begin with some simple sun salutations to awaken the physical body, then move into an asana sequence to relax any tension and oxygenate areas of inflexibility. If you don't have time for a full-sequenced class, a series of sun salutations will be enough to instil a connection with your physical body.

MORNING PRANAYAMA

Following your physical asana practice, each morning you will practise pranayama to settle your internal dialogue and quieten the mind.

Have you ever noticed that when you are feeling anxious, angry or unhappy your breathing pattern is fast, uneven and shallow? But when you are happy or relaxed, your breathing becomes calm and composed? This is because pranayama settles the mind and helps lead you into your meditation.

Please follow the instructions for each breathing exercise as outlined in the daily plan and refer back to page 11 when asked.

DAILY CHAKRA MEDITATION

Try to stay in silence and avoid talking to anyone before you begin if possible. Find a comfortable place which is quiet and peaceful. Wear something warm, light a candle or use dimmed lighting if indoors. Sitting in front of a window with natural light, taking in the view is my preferred indoor space, but sitting on the earth outdoors in nature is always the best place to meditate.

MORNING ROUTINE

After your yoga practice, it is time to get ready for the day ahead. On each day I have outlined your chakra elixir. This is a tonic to your body and an awakening signal to your chakra. Follow these morning rituals and then enjoy your elixir before your breakfast. The elixir should be no more than 90ml (3fl oz/ 6 tablespoons). Follow the recipe to make your chakra elixir each day by referring to the page in the recipe section indicated.

1. Rehydrate. Before doing anything else, pour yourself a cup of tepid to warm water and add a slice of fresh lemon and a tablespoon of raw apple cider vinegar to wake up your liver and digestive system.

2. Set your intention for the day ahead. Jump in the shower and go about getting dressed and packed for the day. While you are in the shower, I recommend coming up with your intention for the day. An intention is more than a wish; it is a direction you work towards, like a goal. But instead of focusing on the result, you focus on the path towards getting there. Stay open to infinite possibilities and always state your intention in the positive. For example, use language such as: 'I will be peaceful and balanced in every situation.' Once you have decided on your intention, surrender it to the universe and enjoy the freedom of not having to try to control everything in your life.

3. Take your morning elixir. It's important to take this on an empty stomach, as it should feel like a shock to your system. Resist the urge to wash it down with water; instead, try to enjoy the sensations as it enters your body and wakes up your senses.

4. Breakfast. Hopefully you will be able to enjoy your breakfast in the comfort of your own home, but if not, then try to enjoy it while seated at a table and without rushing.

DAILY CHAKRA TASK

Your daily task can be completed at any time during the day. You may like to involve others in the task also. Adapt as you see fit.

AFTERNOON PRANAYAMA

These breathing exercises are best performed during your lunch break or during the day while you are taking a short walk somewhere. If you are at home, take a short walk around the block or enjoy a walk around your house while breathing and meditating at the same time. Please follow the instructions for each breathing exercise as outlined on page 11.

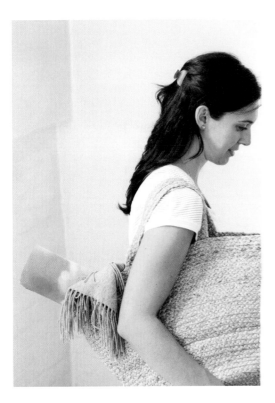

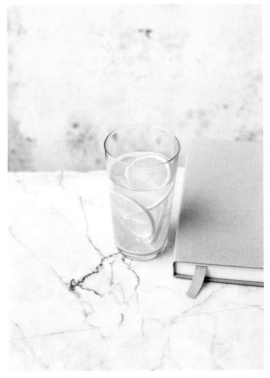

DAILY CHAKRA AFFIRMATION

Before ending your meditation, say out loud four times the daily affirmation outlined for you. This will help you balance the particular chakra and be a mantra for you to keep coming back to if you feel stressed or imbalanced during your day. Write it down and take it with you, so you can always connect back to it.

DAILY WATER INTAKE

If you struggle to drink water during the day, I recommend setting three repeating daily reminders on your phone at three-hour intervals, which will let you know its time to drink up. They should start at 10AM and run through until 4PM. Carry in your bag or have on your desk a 500ml (17fl oz) glass bottle of water and challenge yourself to drink it within that three-hour period. If you prefer to drink tea, then substitute the water bottle for 4–5 cups of herbal tea during the day. These count towards your daily water intake as long as the tea does not contain any caffeine or sweetener.

DAY 1 : ROOT CHAKRA

ROOT | THRIVE | MULADHARA

On day one of the lifestyle plan, we will be focusing on the root chakra, located at the base of the spine. The root chakra (Muladhara) is responsible for your sense of safety and security on this earthly journey. The word muladhara breaks down into two Sanskrit words: *mula* meaning 'root', and *adhara*, which means 'support' or 'base.' Balancing the root chakra creates the solid foundation for opening the chakras above. Imagine that you're laying the foundation for a house in which you're going to live for a long time. A solid foundation embedded in firm soil will provide the stability you need to create a home filled with joy for years to come.

This chakra anchors us into our bodies, the physical world and the earth. In the same way a plant cannot survive without roots, neither can the psyche of a human being. Our 'roots' represent where we have come from, the earth, the womb, our ancestors and family, and our personal history. Our roots can be seen as the way our system plugs into the larger system of the planet, which is our source. The elements we need for physical survival and health all come from the earth in various forms – the foods we eat, the things we touch and see, the water we drink, the air we breathe and the sounds we hear.

The root chakra is comprised of whatever provides stability in your life. This includes your basic needs such as food, water, shelter and safety, as well as your more emotional needs, such family, security and a sense of belonging. When these needs are met, you feel grounded and safe, and tend to worry less day to day.

DAILY PLAN

WAKE WITH THE SUNRISE
(See page 13.)

BODY SCAN
On day one, pay particular attention to the structural form of your body. How do your joints, muscles and skeletal system feel today? Do you feel strong or weak in your body?

ASANA PRACTICE
Associated with the element earth, representing physical and emotional grounding, root chakra poses such as *tadasana* (mountain pose) and *virabhadrasana* (warrior pose) often focus on the feet to help ground you, as well as stretch and strengthen the legs. They're designed to bring you back to your body, to the earth and a sense of safety, security and stillness.

When your hamstrings are tight, the contraction creates a sense that you're constantly prepared to run away. *Uttanasana* (standing forward bend) and *janu sirsasana* (head-to-knee pose) can help to create calmness, patience and a willingness to slow down and stay in one place. When you strengthen the quadriceps and open your hamstrings, you renew your confidence and commitment to the next steps in your life's journey. As you can lean into these poses and ease your fears, you may learn to trust the earth and your body.

Finishing your practice with peaceful restorative poses, such as *supta baddha konasana* (reclining bound angle pose), *savasana* (corpse pose) and *balasana* (child's pose), settles an overactive mind and encourages you to surrender to gravity. By the end of the practice, you will feel at home in your body and more prepared for the challenges that may await you in the day.

MORNING PRANAYAMA

Breathing Exercise 1 – The Breath of Life
(see page 11).

THRIVE MEDITATION
(10–20 MINUTES)

Begin by taking a moment to sit and get grounded.

Place your hands on your thighs, palms down, and begin breathing deeply and slowly. Breathe audibly at first, then allow your breathing to become increasingly quieter. Bring awareness to the weight of your seat and rise tall in your spine. Continue breathing evenly between the inhale and exhale until you feel present and steady at your core.

Now ask yourself these questions and allow yourself enough time between moving onto the next question to sit with your answer and analyse how the answer makes you feel.

1. How do I define myself?
2. Who am I today?
3. Do I feel safe and secure?
4. Where do I feel most at home?
5. Who are the people in my 'tribe'?

THRIVE ELIXIR

Beetroot & Ginger Elixir (page 178)

THRIVE TASK

Today's task is to de-clutter your life and let go of three items you no longer feel you identify with or that do not bring you joy. Recycle these items by taking them to a charity store or passing them onto someone who will use them instead.

AFTERNOON PRANAYAMA

Breathing Exercise 2 – A Walking Meditation
(page 11).

RECIPE PLAN

Breakfast
Apple & Raspberry Bircher
Strawberry Fields Oaty Smoothie
Creamy Vanilla Chia Pudding
Coconut Dream Hibiscus & Berry Smoothie

Lunch
Fennel, Beetroot, Balsamic & Orange Salad
Thrive Gratitude Bowl

Dinner
Celeriac 'Pasta' Lasagna
Harvest Hasselbacks

THRIVE AFFIRMATION

Keep making this affirmation through the day:

I AM CENTRED AND GROUNDED.

I AM AT PEACE WITH THE MATERIAL WORLD AROUND ME AND I KNOW THE UNIVERSE PROTECTS ME.

I AM FULL OF LIFE ENERGY AND ETERNALLY SAFE.

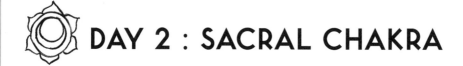

DAY 2 : SACRAL CHAKRA

SACRAL | HONOUR | SVADHISTHANA

On day two of the lifestyle plan we will be focusing on the second chakra, Svadhisthana, also known as the creativity and sexual chakra. It is located above the pubic bone and below the navel. The word *svadhisthana* can be translated as the 'dwelling place of the self', and the element of the second chakra is water, which equals cohesiveness. A balanced second chakra leads to feelings of wellness, abundance, pleasure and joy. When this chakra is out of balance, a person may experience emotional instability, fear of change, sexual dysfunction, depression or addiction.

You can open this chakra with creative expression and by honouring your body. This creativity can be expressed as procreation, but the second chakra energy is certainly not limited to bringing family into this world. When we cook, bake or garden, we are creating. We create when we find a new solution to an old problem. Any time we take raw materials, physical or mental, and transform them into something new, we use our creative energy.

DAILY PLAN

WAKE WITH THE SUNRISE
(See page 13.)

BODY SCAN

On day two pay particular attention to your digestive system and sexual function. Do you feel bloated or hungry? Do you have a dry or pungent mouth? How is your libido? Have you felt sexually aroused recently? Do you feel excited to start your day knowing you have the whole day ahead of you to bring joy to your life and those around you?

ASANA PRACTICE

Along with the sacral chakra at the pelvis, the other even-numbered chakras (the fourth, at the heart, and the sixth, at the third eye) are connected with the 'feminine' energies of relaxation and openness. These chakras exercise our rights to feel, to love, and to see. Odd-numbered chakras, found in the legs and feet at the root chakra, solar plexus, throat, and crown of the head, are connected with the 'masculine' energies of applying our will on the world, asserting our rights to have, to ask, to speak, and to know. The odd-numbered, masculine chakras tend to move energy through our systems, pushing it out into the world and creating warmth and heat. The even-numbered, feminine chakras cool things down, attracting energy inward.

Here in the feminine sacral chakra, asanas help us with adaptability and receptivity. The leg position in *gomukhasana* (cow face pose), forward bending with the legs in the first stage of eka pada *rajakapotasana* (pigeon pose), *baddha konasana* (bound angle pose), *upavistha konasana* (open angle pose), and other hip and groin openers all provide freedom of movement in the pelvis. These hip and groin openers should never be forced, for they require the subtle feminine touch of sensitivity and surrender.

Trikonasana (triangle pose), *bhujangasana* (cobra pose), *natarajasana* (dancers or Shiva pose) and *badhakonasana* (butterfly pose) are also great sacral chakra poses for inner confidence and healthy desires.

MORNING PRANAYAMA
Ida Nadi
This left nostril breathing exercise will help to open up the second chakra. Simply close your right nostril with the first two fingers of

your right hand and inhale and exhale deeply through your left nostril only. Repeat for 8 to 10 breaths.

HONOUR MEDITATION (10–20 MINUTES)

Begin by taking a moment to allow your belly to settle.

Place your hands on your thighs, palms down, and begin bringing attention to your breath. Sense your belly opening and receiving the gentle wisdom of your emotional body with each breath. Pay attention and honour the feelings as they cycle through your consciousness. These sensations are sacred messages of body intelligence intended to keep you aware of what needs your attention and bring you back home within yourself.

Now ask yourself these questions and allow yourself enough time between moving onto the next question to sit with your answer and analyze how the answer makes you feel.

1. How can I honour myself today?
2. How can I bring more pleasure and joy into my life today?
3. Do I feel there is fluidity and ease in my life?
4. What change may I be resisting?
5. How will I allow myself to be creative today?

HONOUR ELIXIR

Pink Grapefruit, Lemon & Ginger Elixir (page 178).

HONOUR TASK

Today's task is to enjoy at least 30 minutes of creativity. This could be via the media of cooking, drawing, colouring, writing, gardening, painting or photography. The objective is to allow self-expression through something creative to help connect you to yourself and your inner passions.

AFTERNOON PRANAYAMA

Breathing Exercise 3 – Walking into Gratitude (page 11).

RECIPE PLAN

Breakfast
Papaya & Raspberry Smoothie Bowl
Coconut & Mango Yoghurt Breakfast Bircher
Spiced Maple, Pecan & Orange Granola
Spelt Pancakes

Lunch
Mango, Mint, Coconut & Chilli Salad
Tempeh Satay Skewers

Dinner
Squash & Lentil Korma
Sweet Potato, Vine Tomato, Halloumi & Kale Tray Bake
Squash, Sage & Spelt Risotto
Stuffed Whole Squash

HONOUR AFFIRMATION

Keep making this affirmation through the day:

I AM ALIVE, CONNECTED AND AWARE.

I EMBRACE PLEASURE AND ABUNDANCE.

I GIVE MYSELF PERMISSION TO ENJOY THE DAY AND BE CREATIVE TODAY.

THE SWEETNESS OF LIFE FLOWS THROUGH ME AND I RADIATE ITS JOY.

DAY 3: SOLAR PLEXUS CHAKRA

SOLAR PLEXUS | RADIANCE | MANIPURA

On day three of the lifestyle plan we will be focusing on the third chakra, the solar plexus Manipura, which means 'lustrous gem'. Located around the navel, in the area of the solar plexus and up to the breastbone, this chakra is a source of personal power. It governs self-esteem, warrior energy and the power of transformation. The Manipura chakra also controls metabolism and digestion. When you feel self-confident, have a strong sense of purpose and are self-motivated, your third chakra is open and healthy. If your third chakra is out of balance, you can suffer from low self-esteem, have difficulty making decisions, and may have anger or control issues. When you have clear goals, desires and intentions, you can move forward to achieve them. Each small step you take while honouring the larger intention helps to strengthen your third chakra.

DAILY PLAN

WAKE WITH THE SUNRISE
(See page 13.)

BODY SCAN
On day three pay particular attention to your energy levels. Do you feel like you have the energy needed to go about your daily tasks? Do you breathe deeply or is your breathing shallow? How does your stomach feel? Are you bloated, hungry or nauseous?

ASANA PRACTICE
Third chakra poses fan the flames of your inner fire and restore vitality. Practise *surya namaskar* (sun salutations), abdominal strengtheners like *navasana* (boat pose), *ardha navasana* (half boat pose), and *urdhva prasarita padasana* (leg lifts), warrior poses and twists. Restorative, passive backbends, such as *setu bandhasana* (bridge pose), which cool off the belly's fire, can act as calming agents for the excessive energy in the third chakra. Excessive energy may manifest in hatred, anger, perfectionism and an emphasis on power and status.

MORNING PRANAYAMA
Bhastrika Breath
Improve both digestion and metabolism with the *bhastrika* breath, which may take some time to get used to, but once you do, you will enjoy the fire it builds within you each morning. Sit comfortably with the spine tall and the shoulders relaxed. Start by taking a few deep breaths in and out of your nose with the lips closed. Then, forcefully inhale through your nose, while inflating your lower abdomen and follow this by forcefully exhaling through your nose, while pressing your lower abdomen towards the spine. Use a one-second count on the inhalation and a one-second count on the exhalation at a rapid pace. You will feel like you're getting an abdominal workout. Try for ten repetitions, then work it up to 15 or 20. After you're finished, you will feel a tingling or glowing feeling around the navel.

RADIANCE MEDITATION (10–20 MINUTES)
Begin by taking time to sit quietly, hands on your thighs, palms up, arms straight and relaxed, index fingers and thumbs touching.

Allow your spine to rise tall to create a sense of readiness. Let your breathing rise and fall naturally, bringing awareness to the space just below your heart. Feel it energized and filled with warming energy.

Feel confidence rising within you as you answer the following questions:

1. Do I feel in harmony with my visual surroundings?
2. Is my integrity in check? How could I improve my integrity?
3. Do I express my identity without imposing my will upon others?
4. Do I respect other people's differences?
5. How do I exert my willpower?

RADIANCE ELIXIR

Lemon, Pineapple, Turmeric & Black Pepper Elixir (page 178).

RADIANCE TASK

Set a goal that you've been putting off for some time. Break it down into small steps, and give yourself a timeline to complete each step. The idea is not to be rigid, but to get moving and to take action so that you can make a tangible step forwards towards your goal today. The size of the goal doesn't matter. All that matters is to start moving towards it.

AFTERNOON PRANAYAMA

Breathing Exercise 2 – A Walking Meditation (page 11).

RECIPE PLAN

Breakfast
Orange Blossom Labneh
Sweet Mango & Turmeric Porridge Bowl

Lunch
A Really Good Fattoush
Grilled Lettuce, Corn & Black Bean Chop Salad
Turmeric Burrito
Pearl Barley, Turmeric & Carrot Kimchi Salad

Dinner
Sicilian Green Olive Polenta Pizzas
Golden Cauliflower Chickpea Stew
Soft Shell Tacos with Corn Fritters

RADIANCE AFFIRMATION

Keep making this affirmation through the day:

I AM CONFIDENT IN ALL THAT I DO;

I RESPECT MYSELF AT ALL TIMES AND STAND UP FOR MYSELF WHEN NECESSARY.

I CHOOSE HEALTH, HEALING AND HAPPINESS.

I ACT WITH COURAGE AND STRENGTH AND HAVE INFINITE ENERGY TO LIVE A WONDERFUL LIFE.

DAY 4 : HEART CHAKRA

HEART | LOVE | ANAHATA

The fourth chakra is at the centre of the seven chakras with three below and three above. This is the area where physical and spiritual energies meet. The fourth chakra, also referred to as the heart chakra, is located at the centre of the chest and includes the heart, cardiac plexus, thymus gland, lungs and breasts. It also rules the lymphatic system. The Sanskrit word for the fourth chakra is Anahata, which means 'unstuck' or 'unhurt'. The name implies that beneath the hurts and grievances of past experiences lies a pure and spiritual place where no hurt exists.

When your heart chakra is open, you are flowing with love and compassion, you are quick to forgive, and you accept others and yourself. A closed heart chakra can give way to grief, anger, jealousy, fear of betrayal, and hatred towards yourself and others.

DAILY PLAN

WAKE WITH THE SUNRISE
(See page 13.)

BODY SCAN
On day four pay particular attention to your circulation. Do you feel overly hot or cold? If you are a premenstrual female, do your breasts hurt? Do you feel short of breath or have a cough? Do you have palpitations?

ASANA PRACTICE
Asanas that enliven the heart chakra include passive chest openers in which we arch gently over a blanket or bolster; shoulder stretches, such as the arm positions of *gomukhasana* (cow face pose) and *garudasana* (eagle pose) and backbends, such as *marjariasana* (cat pose) and *ustrasana* (camel pose). Being an even-numbered, feminine chakra, the heart centre naturally yearns to release and let go. Doing backbends develops the trust and surrender we need to open the heart fully.

When we feel fearful, there is no room for love, and our bodies show contraction. When we choose love, the fear melts away and yoga practice takes on a joyful quality. In many backbend poses, the heart is positioned higher than the head. It's wonderfully refreshing to let the mind drop away from the top position and instead allow the body to lead with the heart.

Some signs that the heart chakra is over-powering your life can include co-dependency, possessiveness, jealousy, heart disease and high blood pressure. For these symptoms, forward bends such as *uttanasana* (forward bending pose) are the best antidote, because they are grounding and foster introspection.

MORNING PRANAYAMA
Breathing Exercise 1 – The Breath of Life (page 11).

LOVE MEDITATION (10–20 MINUTES)
Find a comfortable position where your back is fully supported. Try lying down completely or with your feet up a wall; or sitting in a chair, or on the ground with your back against the wall.

Once you have found your place, pay attention to your breath. Notice your body: where is there spaciousness? Where is there tension? Move your attention to your back and its contact with the chair, wall or floor. Allow yourself to feel supported. Holding this support in your body's awareness, turn your breath and attention towards your heart space. Is there fear? Is there hope? Is there a bit of both? Just notice. Once again, release into the support against your back as deeply as you are able. As you do, is there room to relax and soften your heart space? And to create more space on the exhale? Explore without judgment. When you are ready, begin to expand your attention to the room around you, feeling only love for everything you see.

Now ask yourself these questions:

1. How does love manifest itself in my life?
2. How do I offer my own being self-love?
3. Who do I need to forgive?
4. How do I withhold my love?
5. How can I foster the energy flow of love in my life so that it floods my entire life?

LOVE ELIXIR
Apple & Wheatgrass Elixir (page 179).

LOVE TASK
A great way to feel grateful for what we have is to start giving. Your task on day four is to find a way to put giving into action. Try a random act of kindness, offer your time, or simply give someone who needs it a hug. Give it a go; you've got absolutely nothing to lose and everything to gain!

AFTERNOON PRANAYAMA
Breathing Exercise 3 – Walking into Gratitude (page 11).

RECIPE PLAN

Breakfast
Green Glow Overnight Oats
Coconut Cashew Cream Cheese Crostini
Green Smoothie Bowl

Lunch
Sprouted Mung Bean Slaw
Courgette Ribbon, White Bean Smash
  & Pesto Bruschetta
Five-Minute Pea & Mint Soup

Dinner
Flaxseed Linguine
Spring Green Saag Curry
Ricotta, Courgette & Parmesan Fritters
Kimchi-Marinated Kale Buddha Bowl

LOVE AFFIRMATION

Keep making this affirmation through the day:

I AM KIND AND LOVING TO MYSELF.

I ALLOW LOVE TO FILL ME UP AND GUIDE ME IN ALL MY ACTIONS.

I AM ABLE TO LET GO OF THE PAST, TO FORGIVE OTHERS AND MYSELF.

I AM LOVE, I EMBODY LOVE AND I SEE IT ALL AROUND ME.

DAY 5 : THROAT CHAKRA

THROAT | TRUTH | VISHUDDHA

The fifth chakra, Vishuddha, is the first of the three spiritual chakras. In the area of the throat, it governs the anatomical regions of the thyroid, parathyroid, jaw, neck, mouth, tongue and larynx. To be open and aligned in the fifth chakra is to speak and listen, and express yourself using a higher form of communication.

Work on the lower chakras will help prepare you for this level of communication. For example, when you align the first and second chakras, it helps with overcoming fear. Opening the third chakra helps you to feel your personal power and have the confidence to express yourself. Knowing what's in your heart comes when you align the fourth chakra. Then, when it comes to verbalizing your needs, desires and opinions, you're better able to determine how to be truthful to yourself and others.

Authentic expression is not something that comes easily. There's a delicate dance between saying what you mean and staying tactful or diplomatic. Often it's easier to say what another person may want to hear instead of speaking your truth. Fear of not being accepted, or judgment of others may hinder your ability to express yourself truthfully.

DAILY PLAN

WAKE WITH THE SUNRISE
(See page 13.)

BODY SCAN

On day five pay particular attention to your throat area. Do you have a sore throat? How does your neck feel? Does your jaw feel tight? Does your mouth feel dry? Does your tongue feel swollen or coated? Does your speech come easily or does your voice feel coarse?

ASANA PRACTICE

The throat chakra resonates with our inner truth and helps us find a personal way to convey our voice to the outside world. The rhythm of music, creativity of dance, vibration of singing, and the communication we make through writing and speaking are all fifth-chakra ways to express ourselves. During this practice I like to turn some music on and enjoy singing along and having a boogie.

Deficient energy in this chakra leads to neck stiffness, shoulder tension, teeth grinding, throat ailments, and possibly an underactive thyroid. Excessive talking, an inability to listen, hearing difficulties, stuttering, and an overactive thyroid are all related to excessiveness in this chakra. Depending on the ailments, neck stretches and shoulder openers including *ustrasana* (camel pose), *setu bandha sarvangasana* (bridge pose), *sarvangasana* (shoulder stand) and *halasana* (plough pose) can help balance the energy flow in the fifth chakra.

MORNING PRANAYAMA

Lion's Breath
Kneel on the floor and cross the front of your right ankle over the back of your left. Your feet will point out to the sides. Sit back so your perineum snuggles down onto your top right heel. Then press your palms firmly against your knees. Fan your palms and splay your fingers, like the sharpened claws of a lion.

Take a deep inhalation through your nose. Then simultaneously open your mouth wide and stretch out your tongue. Curling the tip of your tongue down towards your chin, open your eyes wide, contract the muscles on the front of your throat, and exhale slowly through your mouth with a distinct 'ha' sound. Your breath should pass over the back of your throat. Breathe in through your nose and repeat the lion's breath exhalation five times. Then change the cross of your legs and repeat.

TRUTH MEDITATION (10–20 MINUTES)

Take a cleansing breath in and breathe out the tension in your body. Allow your breathing to fall into its own natural rhythm. Don't try to control it in any way – just observe it as you breathe in relaxation and breathe out tension. Bring your attention to your throat area. Imagine a lovely little sky-blue light there swirling around like a little whirlpool. Try to notice how it feels, how it looks. Try to get a sense of how it is functioning – can you feel any tingling? What thoughts are popping into your head? Is it swirling and moving? What speed is it? Does it feel fast or slow? Is it a little light or a big light?

As you focus on this spinning blue wheel, focus on your truest expressions and answer these questions:

1. Do I speak what is in my heart freely, openly and truthfully?
2. Do I express my authentically through my words?
3. Do I feel listened to by those around me?
4. Do I hold back from speaking my truth? When?
5. Do I fear pain from people's words? Why?

TRUTH ELIXIR

Spirulina & Strawberry Elixir (page 179).

TRUTH TASK

Sing! Singing is an amazing throat-chakra cleanser, so sing your favourite song out loud and enjoy opening up your voice to those high notes.

AFTERNOON PRANAYAMA

Breathing Exercise 2 – A Walking Meditation (see page 11).

RECIPE PLAN

Breakfast
Poached Pear & Rhubarb Compote
  & Pistachio Crumble
Blackberry, Buckwheat & Stewed
  Apple Porridge
Raisin Bread French Toast
Asparagus & Goat's Curd Socca

Lunch
Beetroot, Spinach & Goat's Cheese Galette
Chickpea 'Tofu' Chips
Horseradish, Watercress, Celeriac
  & Apple Salad

Dinner
Green Bean & Artichoke Quinoa Salad

TRUTH AFFIRMATION

Keep making this affirmation through the day:

I SPEAK MY TRUTH AND EXPRESS MYSELF WITH CLARITY AND CONFIDENCE.

I LIVE AUTHENTICALLY.

DAY 6 : THIRD-EYE CHAKRA

THIRD EYE | INTUITION | AJNA

The sixth chakra, Ajna, is in the area of the third eye, which is found in the space between the eyebrows. This is your centre of intuition. It encompasses the pituitary gland, eyes, head and lower part of the brain. A spiritual chakra which means 'beyond wisdom', Ajna leads you to an inner knowledge that will guide you if you let it.

It's this intuition and wholeness that allows us to look at our physical body as an integrated whole. Instead of limbs and organs we are able to take an holistic view of each and every aspect of our physical selves and bring ourselves to oneness.

This is where we can find an understanding of our true health. No longer concerned by mere symptoms, our minds are able to process and see the body as a complete system. Reaching a deeper understanding of our health means we are able finally to listen to what our bodies need and act accordingly.

DAILY PLAN

WAKE WITH THE SUNRISE
(See page 13.)

BODY SCAN

On day six pay particular attention to your eyes, head and brain. Do you have a headache or dry eyes? How is your disposition? Do you feel happy, irritated or particularly moody? Are you more tired than usual? Do you feel cold? Do you feel hormonal?

ASANA PRACTICE

When the third eye is over-stimulated, you may experience headaches, hallucinations, nightmares and difficulty concentrating. At the opposite end of the scale, when the third eye is deficient in energy, you may experience poor memory, eye problems and difficulty recognizing patterns, and you may struggle to visualize or tap into your imagination.

Poses that support the Ajna chakra are supported forward bends, adding an extra bolster or blanket to press upon and stimulate the third-eye area, or simply drop into *balasana* (child's pose) and rest your forehead on your mat.

Other poses to help connect to your inner self include *adho mukha svanasana* (downward facing dog), *vajrasan* (thunderbolt pose) and *anjaneyasana* (low lunge pose).

MORNING PRANAYAMA
Brahmari
A great breathing exercise to help balance the third-eye chakra is known as *brahmari* or the bee breath. To do this exercise, sit comfortably, with your back tall and shoulders relaxed. Start by taking a few natural breaths, and close your eyes. Then, keeping your lips lightly sealed, inhale through your nostrils. Exhaling, make the sound of the letter 'm', essentially a humming sound. Sustain the sound until you need to inhale. Then repeat: inhale through your nose, then hum like a buzzing bee as you exhale. Continue by inhaling, then exhaling with this sound for 15 breaths.

INTUITION MEDITATION
(10–20 MINUTES)

Begin to tune into your intuitive power – your ability to perceive, know and experience with all your senses beyond the realm of the physical and into the realm of the divine. Breathe deeply into your lower abdomen, letting it fill up with the light of the divine that is all around you. Breathe in and breathe out. As you exhale, let go of any tension, worry or struggle, any energy that is not yours. Breathe in the divine light that is all around you and as you breathe out, feel yourself relaxing deeply, entering fully into this present space and time, becoming aware and becoming present.

Focus on your breath, and as you take in another deep breath through your nose, breathe air into your lower abdomen, filling yourself up with the light of the divine. As you exhale, tune into your energetic field, which is infused with the divine light all around you. Imagine your energy as a sort of hourglass shape, receiving with open arms the light of the divine, intuitive guidance, infinite wisdom, wellbeing, healing and love, which flow down into your being from above. Imagine the middle of your hourglass energetic form strong, stable and present.

Visualize your core energy filled with light, helping you to increase your awareness, to be fully present at this time. Then imagine the light flowing out and down, grounding you to the Earth. Follow this light down to the core of Earth and then you will feel your oneness with the divine.

Now ask yourself these questions:

1. Do I trust myself?
2. Do I allow myself to dream and visualize my future?
3. Do I enjoy spending time in my dreams?
4. How is my intuition a part of my daily life?
5. What does wisdom mean to me?

INTUITION ELIXIR
Blackberry, Ginger & Aloe Vera Elixir (page 179).

INTUITION TASK
On day six spend some time in visualization. Imagine a goal you would like to achieve, then I want you to find a comfortable place to sit and begin to visualize what it would feel like to wake up in your body once you have reached that goal. Walk around in your imagination as

if you are living the life you visualize, with your successes and dreams realized.

AFTERNOON PRANAYAMA
Breathing Exercise 3 – Walking into Gratitude (see page 11).

RECIPE PLAN

Breakfast
Hazelnut & Cacao Porridge
Pick-Me-Up Cacao Granola
Chai-Spiced Porridge

Lunch
Pistachio & Freekeh Tabouleh
Nut Cheese with Chilled Blackberry Soup
Turmeric Cauliflower, Carrot & Chickpea Salad
Ricotta, Roasted Grapes & Thyme Bruschetta

Dinner
Roasted Tomato & Spinach Dhal
Courgetti Puttanesca
Radicchio, Grape & Balsamic Tray Bake
Teriyaki Cauliflower Bites

INTUITION AFFIRMATION

Keep making this affirmation through the day:

I AM CONNECTED TO AND HONOUR MY INTUITION ALWAYS.

IT IS SAFE FOR ME TO SEE THE TRUTH AND TRANSFORM.

DAY 7 : CROWN CHAKRA

CROWN | CONNECTION | SAHASWARA

The seventh and final chakra is located at the crown of the head. Sahaswara is our source of enlightenment and spiritual connection to all that is. It is a connection to our higher selves, to every being on the planet, and to the divine energy that creates everything in the universe.

The crown chakra is the ultimate point where all is pure, simple and intentional. The prime activity of the seventh chakra is to derive meaning. This is where the element of thought is witnessed. To arrive at the fully blooming lotus, Sahaswara, our stem needs to be connected all the way to the Earth, with our roots firmly in the ground. Through this connection to all other elements and the Earth, we are able to nourish and bloom, and continue to expand, yet stay connected to where we have come from.

DAILY PLAN

WAKE WITH THE SUNRISE
(See page 13.)

BODY SCAN

On day seven pay particular attention to your dreams. Do you remember what you were just dreaming about? Can you find meaning in your dream? Does your mind feel open and free to wander, or confused and busy? Do you feel connected to your higher self or burdened by life's issues?

ASANA PRACTICE

Excessiveness in this chakra appears as being overly intellectual or possessing a feeling of spiritual or intellectual elitism. Deficient energy manifests as difficulty thinking for yourself, apathy, spiritual scepticism, and materialism. Meditation is the yogic practice best suited to bringing this chakra into balance. Thus *padmasana* (lotus pose) is the expected pose here. The energy of the crown chakra helps us to experience the divine, to be open to a higher or deeper power, allowing the mind to become more present, clear and insightful.

Poses to help you connect to this chakra include *sirsasana* (headstand pose), *matsyasana* (fish pose) and *vriksasana* (tree pose).

MORNING PRANAYAMA
Alternate nostril breathing
Sit comfortably with your spine erect and shoulders relaxed. Keep a gentle smile on your face. Place your left hand on your left knee, palm open to the sky or in *chin mudra* (thumb and index finger gently touching at the tips). Place the tip of your index finger and middle finger of your right hand in between your eyebrows, your ring finger and little finger on your left nostril, and your thumb on the right nostril. We will use the ring finger and little finger to open or close the left nostril and thumb for the right nostril.

Press your thumb down on your right nostril and breathe out gently through your left nostril. Now breathe in through your left nostril, then press your left nostril gently with your ring finger and little finger. Removing your right thumb from your right nostril, breathe out from the right. Breathe in from your right nostril and exhale from your left.

You have now completed one round of alternate nostril breathing. Continue inhaling and exhaling from alternate nostrils. Complete nine rounds. After every exhalation, remember to breathe in from the same nostril from which you exhaled. Keep your eyes closed and keep taking long, deep breaths without force or effort.

CONNECTION MEDITATION (10–20 MINUTES)

Take a cleansing breath in and breathe out any tension. Allow your breathing to fall into its own rhythm, not trying to control it in any way.

Imagine a big, white lotus with its petals closed in the same place as your crown chakra. Look at the lotus and contemplate its shape, colour and texture. As you pay attention, the lotus slowly starts to swirl along with the chakra. One by one the petals of the lotus start to open.

As the first layer flowers, you see uncountable rows of more petals still to open. As every petal opens, the lotus spins faster. You realize that every such opening leads to yet another layer of closed petals. The blooming of the lotus is a process of infinite stages. Now see your seventh chakra spinning with equal strength. The chakra's violet light washes over you and pervades every cell, every pore in your body. Breathe deeply and feel the energy from your crown chakra connecting you to the sky above, the Earth below, and everything in between.

Rest in this awareness and ask yourself:

1. How do I feel when I feel connected to the Earth and the universe around me?
2. How can I easily tune back into this higher-self energy source?
3. Do I see everything around me as one?
4. How can I thank the universe for the profound experience of my life?
5. How can I channel my highest good into my daily life?

CONNECTION ELIXIR

Aloe Vera, Lime & Coconut Elixir (page 179).

CONNECTION TASK

This exercise is simple, but incredibly powerful because it helps you to notice and appreciate seemingly simple elements of your environment in a more profound way. The exercise is designed to connect you with the beauty of the natural environment, something we can easily miss when we are rushing.

1. Choose a natural object from within your immediate environment and focus on it, watching it for a minute or two. This could be a flower or an insect, the clouds or the moon.
2. Don't do anything except notice the thing you are looking at. Simply relax into watching for as long as your concentration allows.
3. Look at this object as if you are seeing it for the first time. Visually explore every aspect of its formation, and allow yourself to be consumed by its presence.
4. Allow yourself to connect with its energy and its purpose within the natural world.

AFTERNOON PRANAYAMA

Breathing Exercise 2 – A Walking Meditation (page 11).

RECIPE PLAN

Breakfast
Bird of Paradise Pear, Ginger & Coconut Milk Smoothie
Summer Love Smoothie

Lunch
Yogi Caesar Salad
Broccoli, Coriander & White Miso Soup
Boneless Gut-Healing Broth

Dinner
Zen Mango, Avocado Courgetti Bowl
Bro-Sushi
Creamy Tarragon, Pea & Spinach Shakshouka

CONNECTION AFFIRMATION

Keep making this affirmation through the day:

I SEE BEYOND MY LIMITING BELIEFS AND ACCEPT MY HUMAN EXPERIENCE FULLY.

I HONOUR MY BODY AS THE TEMPLE THAT NOURISHES MY SOUL.

I AM DIVINELY GUIDED AND INSPIRED.

I AM INFINITE AND BOUNDLESS.

THE YOGA KITCHEN
EATING PRINCIPLES

Once you start to explore the connections between your mind, body and spirit, you inevitably begin to gravitate towards a type of diet that gives you nourishment, energy, lightness and flexibility.

A yogi diet is a balanced diet that ancient yogis believed had a huge influence not only over your physical wellbeing, but also over your thoughts, and ultimately your emotional and spiritual wellbeing. With continued awareness of the body through yoga, you may find that vegetarian and vegan foods become a natural choice. They can help you maintain the same energized, light feeling that you achieve through yoga.

The following six yogi eating principles are my guides to help you maintain a calm and steady mind, while also having the energy for your daily yoga practice and daily tasks. If you can follow and incorporate these principles into your daily life, I promise you will feel happier, healthier and more vibrant.

A PURE 'LIFE FORCE'

Like all living organisms in the universe, the foods we eat possess qualities and energies that affect our mind, body and soul. Yogic foods such as fruits and vegetables, nuts and whole grains are known as sattvic, which simply means 'pure essence'. These foods are considered abundant in chi or prana, the universal life force that gives energy to all beings in both the plant and animal kingdoms.

When we eat a pure diet, the food and life force found in these foods bring us physical strength, clarity for our mind, health and longevity. They calm, purify and lead to a peaceful mind in control of a fit body, with a balanced flow of energy between them leading to a peaceful state where higher consciousness becomes accessible. Enjoying these foods enables us to keep an open mind to all possibilities, think more positively, and be far more kind to ourselves and those around us.

Eating a sattvic diet means we get to enjoy the plant kingdom in its total abundance. Whole, real foods, found in their natural state dance together on our plates, offering their vibrancy to us. Foods that are pure, light, soothing and easily digested become our staples.

There are whole grains beautifully arranged around lots of olive oil and vegetables. There are fresh fruits and natural sugars scattered through meals, offering us the taste of sweet in perfect proportions. Handfuls of nuts and seeds bring texture and healthful benefits, and nothing is too stimulating, yet nor is it boring. This way of eating is vegetarian food alchemy in its most beautiful form.

Go ahead, indulge in the life force of plants!

CONSISTENT ENERGY FLOW

As we step into a yogic way of life and find calmness through sattvic foods, we need to find the balance of energy and fire in our bodies with the addition of rajasic foods. Rajasic foods such as cacao, matcha, turmeric, chilli, ginger and cheeses have less life-force energy than sattvic foods, but they are essential in moderation to help stimulate our body and the mind, giving us the energy to get things done. These foods help push us beyond our normal capabilities, creating energy to go out and reach our goals. They are best eaten in the morning and before noon as they can often disrupt normal cortisol levels and create energy imbalances.

The recipes I have created in the meal planner have the perfect balance of rajasic foods to keep you motivated and energized for life. There are cacao nibs and matcha found in my Pick-Me-Up Cacao Granola (page 143) and Green Glow Overnight Oats (page 100) recipes, Sweet Mango & Turmeric Porridge Bowl (page 82) when warmth and fire are needed, or Asparagus & Goat's Curd Socca (page 128) for a cheesy evening treat.

A HAPPY GUT

Consuming probiotic rich, fermented foods, such as miso and sauerkraut, and drinks, such as kefir and kombucha, will introduce beneficial bacteria into your digestive system. These help maintain a balance of good, healthful bacteria against the bad bacteria, which can inhibit the absorption of all the amazing nutrients we will be eating, cause bloating or give us hazy brain fog.

Eating plenty of prebiotic foods, such as asparagus, banana, oats and apples every day feeds these healthy probiotic bacteria and helps keep our immune systems strong. I have filled the recipes with loads of prebiotic ingredients so you don't have to think about it. You will also find plenty of probiotic recipes, such as Blueberry & Basil Kombucha (page 122) and Apple & Beetroot Sauerkraut (page 50).

CALM THROUGH WATER

We all know that drinking water in an essential daily habit. Staying hydrated helps our muscles recover more quickly post-yoga. It also helps flush out the toxins that we eliminate during a yoga class through twisting, sweating and breathing deeply. Here is an easy way to work out how much water you should drink each day: divide your bodyweight in kilos by 30. This number equals how many litres of clean drinking water you should consume daily. Easy!

In the daily programme section, you will find my helpful instructions and guidance on how to maintain a healthful and regular intake of

water each day. What you won't find, however, is my recommendation for liquids during your meals! Too much liquid with meals can dilute the digestive juices we need to properly break down our food. Therefore, I don't recommend you drink large amounts of any fluid, be it juice, water or tea, for at least 30 minutes before a meal or an hour afterwards.

A little liquid with the meal is okay and a glass of warm water with a squeeze of lemon juice half an hour before a meal may promote secretion of stomach acid, but washing our foods down with water will make it hard for our bodies to digest efficiently. If you follow my daily water intake instructions, you will not only get the right amount of water every day, you will also take care of your digestive system.

MOTHER NATURE

Staying connected and in tune with our bodies within the world around us can be achieved by paying attention to the natural world. Staying in tune with the seasons helps us to reap the benefits Mother Nature intended for us. Here is how to move with the seasons…

During the summer months, life is at its most expansive, fully manifested. The sun is at its zenith, food is abundant, and all plant life is full of vital life force. These are the months when we feel the most vibrant and the light, fresh, sweet foods quench our appetite. Foods are literally bursting with nutrients to give us the energy to enjoy the longer days.

During late summer, we experience a distinct shift, a brief pause between the explosive energy of summer and the quiet descent of autumn. While the days are still hot, evenings turn cooler, the sunsets come a bit earlier and the harvest begins to shift from the delicate juicy foods of summer to the hardier foods of autumn. The earth offers up all of her great abundance, and it is a time when all of life seems to balance. This is when the energy of the seasons starts to revert back to the earth and we retreat within ourselves, taking stock of life.

Once autumn arrives the downwards shift occurs; the light lessens, days grow shorter, and energy descends back into the earth for the dormant cycle. We retreat back to our kitchens for heartier meals and find ourselves searching the back of cupboards for lentils and other grains as our bodies call out for starchy, more filling foods.

Winter is the dormant season, when all life force burrows deep into the bosom of the earth. It is a good time to reflect and replenish so that when spring comes, the gathering energy will burst forth with new growth. The cold weather makes us crave our own internal heating and therefore we reach for warming spices and hot, cosy meals.

Then spring arrives and marks a miraculous burst of energy. We can feel we are part of something bigger as we see Mother Nature play out her tricks and bring everything full circle again. Sap, which is nature's lifeblood, courses through the trees, new life pushes its way up from the depths of the earth, and we are surrounded by a bright sense of renewal and creativity in our lives.

To truly stay in tune with your body, Mother Nature and the seasons, always keep an eye out for how you can adapt and substitute recipes to make them more seasonal. I have offered my suggestions through the meal planner recipes for you.

MINDFUL EATING HABITS

EAT SLOWLY AND WITH AWARENESS

Eating doesn't have to be a race. Taking time to savour and enjoy our food is one of the healthiest things we can do: you are more likely to notice when you are full; you'll chew your food more and so digest it more easily; and you'll probably find yourself noticing flavours you might otherwise have missed.

My top tip to help you slow down is to put your fork down between bites – this will encourage you to chew and appreciate each mouthful individually rather than the bowl or plate as a whole.

ELIMINATE DISTRACTIONS

I'm not one for eating in silence, but I must have picked up a thing or two from my family meal times when Mum would turn off the TV and encourage us to enjoy each other's company and share our daily experiences.

Our daily lives are full of distractions and electronic-free zones are now rare, but by disconnecting from the outside world and bringing focus to our body and food, we limit the potential for stress to impact on our digestion, and honour the food that we have chosen to nourish ourselves with.

My tip here is to turn your phone to silent and leave it outside of the room you are eating in so you won't be tempted to pick it up and distract yourself from your meal.

STOP EATING WHEN YOU'RE FULL

It can take 20 to 30 minutes for the brain to know when the stomach is full, which is why we can sometimes unconsciously overeat. The best way to not overeat is to follow tip number one and eat slowly. This gives your brain a chance to catch up with your body and register the signals to eat the right amount; leaving enough room in our stomach for the food we have eaten to be churned with the digestive juices.

You will get to know your body and decipher the right amount of food for your stomach by following these mindful-eating practices, but in the beginning I recommend serving yourself a half portion. Eat this portion slowly, then allow 20 minutes before deciding how much more you would like to eat. In this way you will be able clearly to assess what your body needs and avoid over-burdening your stomach, making digestion uncomfortable.

CONSIDER THE LIFE CYCLE OF FOOD

Sadly, many of us don't consider where a meal comes from beyond the supermarket packaging.

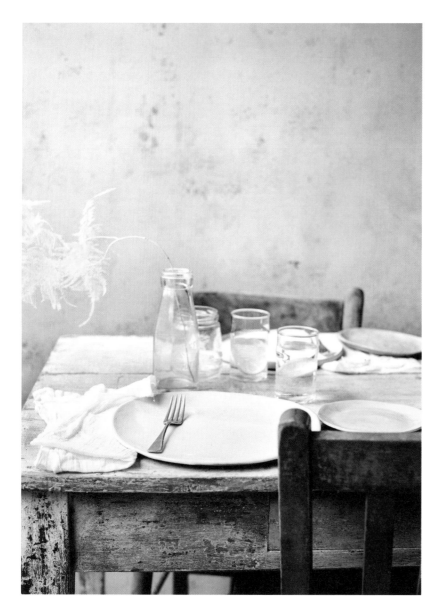

This is a real shame because eating offers an opportunity to connect us more deeply with the natural world and the elements around us.

When we pause to consider all the people involved in the meal that has arrived on our plate – from the loved ones (and yourself) who prepared it, to those who stocked the shelves, to those who planted and harvested the raw ingredients, to those who supported them – it is hard to not feel both grateful and connected to this life cycle.

Be mindful of the water, soil and other elements that were part of your food's creation as you sit down to eat whatever you are eating. It will become effortless to experience gratitude for all the people who gave their energy and the elements of the universe that contributed their share also.

THE PANTRY

These are the ingredients you will find in my yoga kitchen pantry. I use most weekly and a lot of them take pride of place in jars so that the colours and textures inspire me. You will find all these ingredients in supermarkets and all have a long shelf life.

When choosing fruit and veg, be mindful of how they have been grown and transported. I will often choose local over organic if the organic produce has been flown in from another country. To clean your non-organic produce, soak it in a sink full of water with a splash of white vinegar.

PANTRY GOODS

CONDIMENTS, PASTES, LIQUIDS

Chopped tomatoes (cans)
Coconut milk (cans)
Honey
Maple syrup
Raw apple cider vinegar
Tahini paste
Tamari sauce
Tamarind paste
Toasted sesame oil
Vanilla extract
Vegetable stock cubes

LEGUMES, GRAINS, FLOUR, BEANS

Black beans
Buckwheat flour
Buckwheat groats
Butter beans (lima beans)
Cannellini beans
Chickpeas (garbanzo beans) (cans)
Chickpea (gram) flour
Dried green mung beans
Freekeh grains
Polenta
Red kidney beans
Red lentils
Rolled oats
Spelt flour

NUTS, SEEDS, DRIED FRUITS

Almond butter
Brazil nuts
Cacao nibs
Cacao powder
Chia seeds
Coconut flakes
Coconut sugar
Desiccated (dried shredded) coconut
Dried apricots
Dried dates
Dried figs
Goji berries
Ground almonds
Prunes
Pumpkin seeds
Quinoa
Raw almonds
Raw cashews
Raw hazelnuts
Raw shelled pistachios
Raw walnuts
Sunflower seeds

DRIED SPICES

Cumin seeds
Coriander seeds
Curry leaves
Dried chilli (hot pepper) flakes
Dried oregano
Fennel seeds
Garam masala
Ground cinnamon
Ground coriander
Ground cumin
Ground sumac powder
Ground turmeric
Mustard seeds
Sweet smoked paprika

ON THE COUNTER

Black pepper
Coconut oil
Fresh herbs
Olive oil
Sea salt

FRIDGE / FREEZER

Brown & white miso pastes
Coconut water
Edamame beans
Garden peas
Ground flaxseed
Feta cheese
Goat's cheese and curd
Live natural full-fat yoghurt (or alternatives)
Matcha powder (optional)
Milk alternatives: hemp, oat & almond
Mixed berries
Olives
Parmesan cheese
Sauerkraut
Spirulina powder (optional)

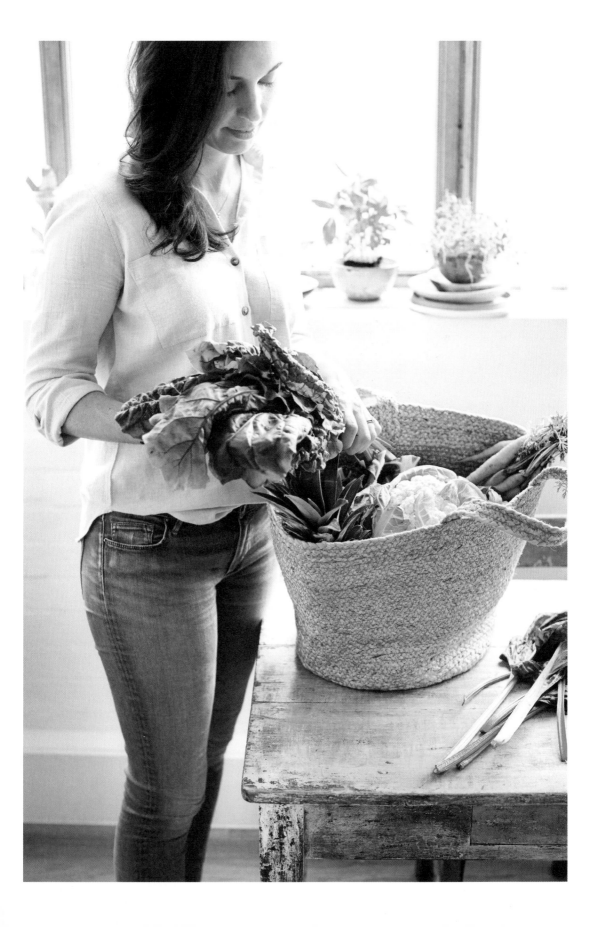

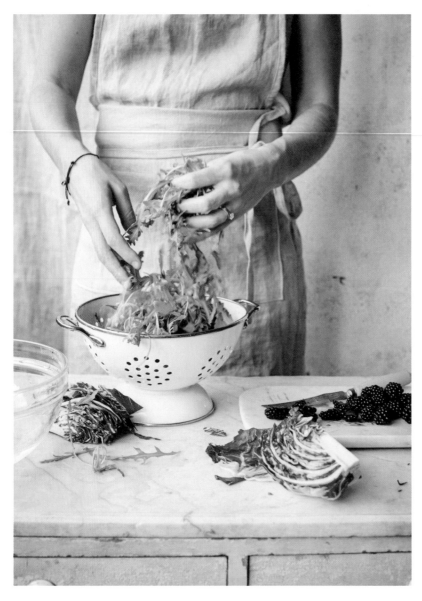

THINK OF THESE RECIPES AS A TEST FOR CREATING INTIMATE,
PLEASURABLE EXPERIENCES FOR YOURSELF. IT MAY SEEM LIKE A
SIMPLE WEEKDAY MEAL, BUT LIGHT SOME CANDLES, LAY OUT THE
TABLE BEAUTIFULLY, FIND A FLOWER TO POP INTO A VASE AND
NURTURE THE SIDE OF YOURSELF THAT ENJOYS SIMPLE FOOD
COOKED REALLY WELL AND EATEN IN SURROUNDINGS THAT FEEL
INTIMATE AND GOOD FOR YOUR SOUL.

THE YOGA KITCHEN
MEAL PLANS

Welcome to your weekly meal planner. Here you will find your daily chakra recipes to complement your lifestyle planner. The meal planner is easy to use; all you have to do is refer to the chakra and choose from the selection of breakfast, lunch and evening meals for that day.

You will find three, well-proportioned meals each day in the meal planner, which you should eat at 4-hour intervals from each other for maximum energy flow during the day. If cooking three recipes is not achievable each day, then there is no reason to stress and feel you are not completing the plan properly. If you can manage just one recipe each day, you will be offering your body a daily gift. As I said earlier, if you miss a day, don't worry; just pick it up the next day. We are human and our path towards a happier, healthier life has no room for perfectionism, so if you follow only part of the programme each day then pat yourself on the back and look forward to the next day.

There are also eight sweet and savoury snack recipes that will boost your energy and I recommend no more than two servings per day.

FOR MAXIMUM ENERGY BEFORE YOUR MORNING CLASS

Avoid eating for at least one hour before your morning yoga practice. The key is to find the balance between nourishing yourself and becoming full. If you eat too much before a class, the heat and energy will go to your digestive tract instead of your practice, and it can become uncomfortable to twist, invert or engage the *bandhas* (muscle contractions).

FOR MAXIMUM ENERGY BEFORE YOUR EVENING CLASS

If you practise in the afternoon or evenings and are famished before class, try snacking on nuts or nut butters and low-acidic and soothing fruits, like bananas, peaches, mangos or berries, at least 20 minutes before class.

ROOT CHAKRA
thrive

Key foods for the root chakra:
RED FOOD: tomato, raspberry, strawberry,
hibiscus, redcurrant
ROOT VEGETABLES: beetroot, parsnip, carrot, sweet
potato, celeriac
FOODS WITH A HIGH INSOLUBLE FIBRE CONTENT:
chia seeds
PROTEIN-RICH FOODS: nuts and pulses
VITAMIN D- AND CALCIUM-RICH FOODS FOR BONE
STRUCTURE: sesame seeds/tahini
GROUNDING SPICES: ginger, cinnamon, clove,
nutmeg, cumin
Enjoy homemade comfort foods and
avoid stimulating foods, such as caffeine
and refined sugars

Bircher has always been my go-to for morning oats during the lighter, brighter summer months. I rarely crave the cosy warmth porridge offers on a sunny summer morning, however this bircher could easily turn into a bowl of warm goodness in the cooler seasons.

If you're making porridge, simply add all the ingredients except the cup of fresh or frozen raspberries into a saucepan and warm through for a few minutes until the oats are cooked and gently simmering as per normal porridge. Once cooked, remove from the heat and stir the mashed raspberries into the porridge and serve topped with chopped raw pistachio crumbs.

APPLE & RASPBERRY BIRCHER
with pistachio confetti (v)

SERVES 2

100g (3½oz/1 cup) rolled oats
½ tablespoon ground cinnamon
240ml (8fl oz/1 cup) almond
    milk, or milk of your choice
1 teaspoon vanilla extract
1 tablespoon maple syrup
2 eating apples, grated
    (keep the skin on)
1 tablespoon sunflower seeds
1 tablespoon pumpkin seeds
125g (4½oz/1 cup) fresh or
    frozen raspberries

TO GARNISH

full-fat, natural yoghurt (vegan
    if necessary)
raw pistachios, roughly chopped
bee pollen (optional for vegans)

Put the oats into a medium mixing bowl, add the cinnamon and stir to combine. Add the milk, vanilla extract and maple syrup and stir again. Now add the grated apples and seeds and stir well. Cover the bowl with cling film (plastic wrap) and refrigerate overnight or for at least 20 minutes. If using frozen raspberries, remove from the freezer and place in a bowl to thaw.

Once the bircher has soaked, uncover and stir to loosen. You may like to add a little water to help loosen the mixture. Mash the fresh or thawed raspberries slightly using a fork. Add the raspberries to the bircher mixture and stir to combine. The bircher will turn a gorgeous light pink colour. Taste and adjust for sweetness and flavour. You may like to add some 0extra cinnamon, raspberries or maple syrup.

Serve the bircher in 2 breakfast bowls with a dollop of yoghurt, a sprinkle of chopped raw pistachio confetti, and a scattering of bee pollen, if wished. Keeps for 3–5 days in the fridge.

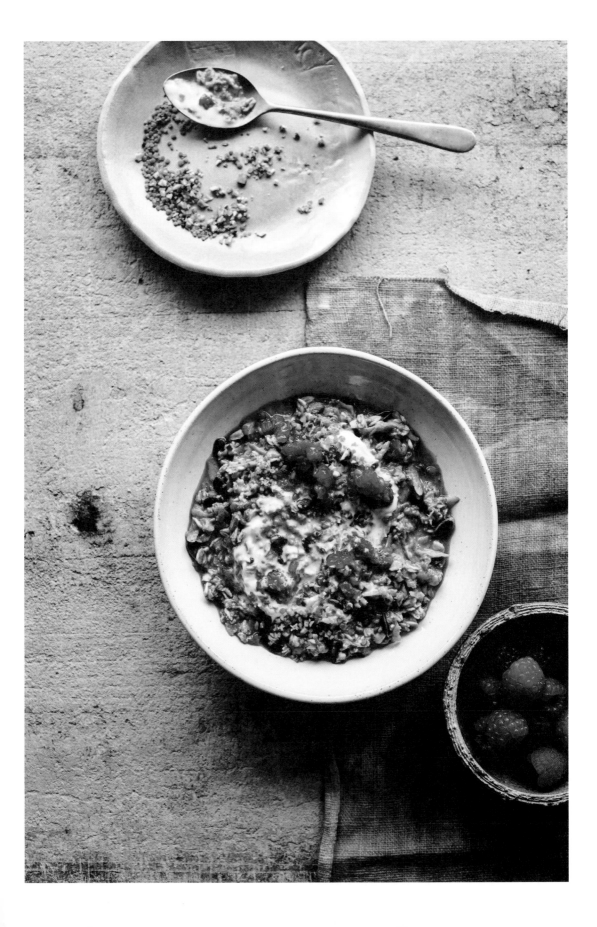

Strawberries make any smoothie classy and this smoothie delivers a gorgeous creamy lightness while still being refreshing. Just what you need after your morning yoga practice. This smoothie will also keep you going as the addition of oats, Greek yoghurt and cashews replenishes your energy and helps you feel fuller for longer.

STRAWBERRY FIELDS OATY SMOOTHIE

SERVES 2

200g (7oz/2 cups) strawberries, hulled and chopped
1 teaspoon vanilla extract
40g (1½oz/scant ½ cup) rolled oats
1 tablespoon raw cashews
120g (4¼oz/½ cup) full-fat, natural coconut or Greek yoghurt
400ml (14fl oz/1¾ cups) oat milk, or alternative milk of your choice
2 tablespoons maple syrup
6–8 ice cubes (optional)

Place the strawberries and vanilla into a blender and blend until smooth. Divide between 2 glasses.

Clean the blender cup, then add the oats, cashews, yoghurt, milk, maple syrup and ice (if using). Blend for 2–3 minutes or until completely smooth. Pour the oat mixture over the strawberry mixture and serve.

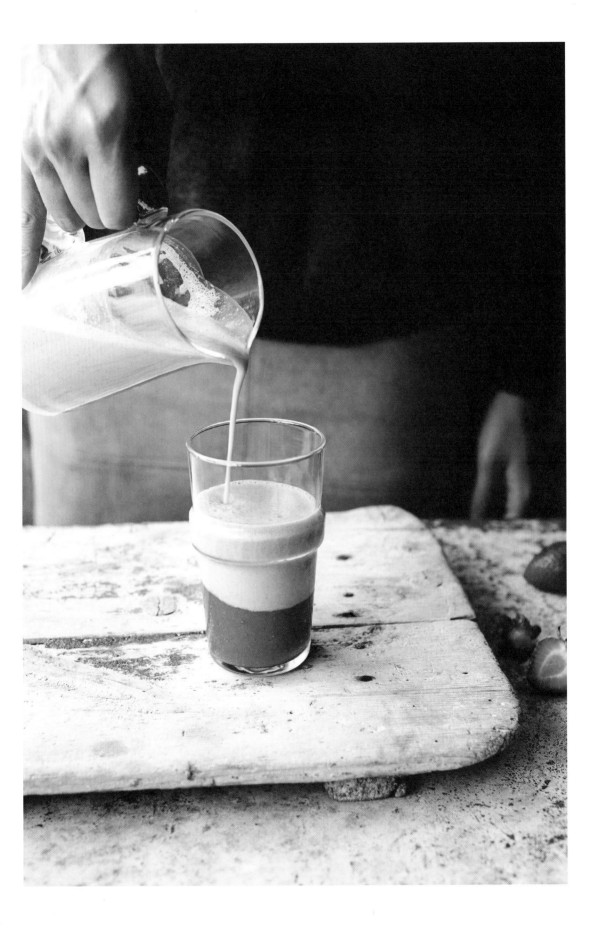

This breakfast is so decadent, it feels like you're having dessert at breakfast time. If strawberries are not in season you can always use frozen strawberries, or fresh or frozen raspberries make a good alternative.

This creamy vanilla and cashew chia cream works with others fruits such as mango purée and passion fruit pulp, so be creative with your seasonal fruits to create the breakfast to suit your taste buds.

CREAMY VANILLA CHIA PUDDING
with strawberry swirls (v)

SERVES 2

200g (7oz/2 cups) strawberries, hulled and quartered

FOR THE VANILLA
CHIA CREAM

30g (1oz/¼ cup) raw cashews or macadamias, soaked in filtered water for 3–4 hours
400ml (14fl oz/1¾ cups) can full-fat coconut milk
2 teaspoons vanilla extract or vanilla bean paste
2 tablespoons maple syrup or 4 dried, pitted dates
75g (2½oz/½ cup) chia seeds

TO GARNISH

full-fat coconut yoghurt
blueberries
raw pistachios, roughly chopped
bee pollen (optional for vegans)

To make the vanilla chia cream, place all the ingredients except the chia seeds into a blender or food processor and blend on high speed for at least 2 minutes or until a smooth liquid has formed and all the nuts and the dates (if using) have been puréed. You're looking for a really smooth consistency.

Pour the cream into a large mixing bowl and whisk in the chia seeds, making sure all the seeds have been evenly distributed in the liquid and there are no lumps. I always use a whisk to ensure I don't miss any chia seeds. Pour the mixture into 2 serving bowls and set aside for at least 20 minutes to allow the chia seeds to absorb the liquid.

Place the strawberries in a shallow bowl and, using the back of a fork, slowly start to mash the strawberries until you have compote-like consistency.

Place a spoonful of the strawberry compote on top of each bowl and then stir into the vanilla chia cream creating a few swirls. Serve with a dollop of yoghurt, a few blueberries, some roughly chopped raw pistachios and some bee pollen, if desired.

Store in the fridge for up to 3 days or in the freezer for longer-term storage.

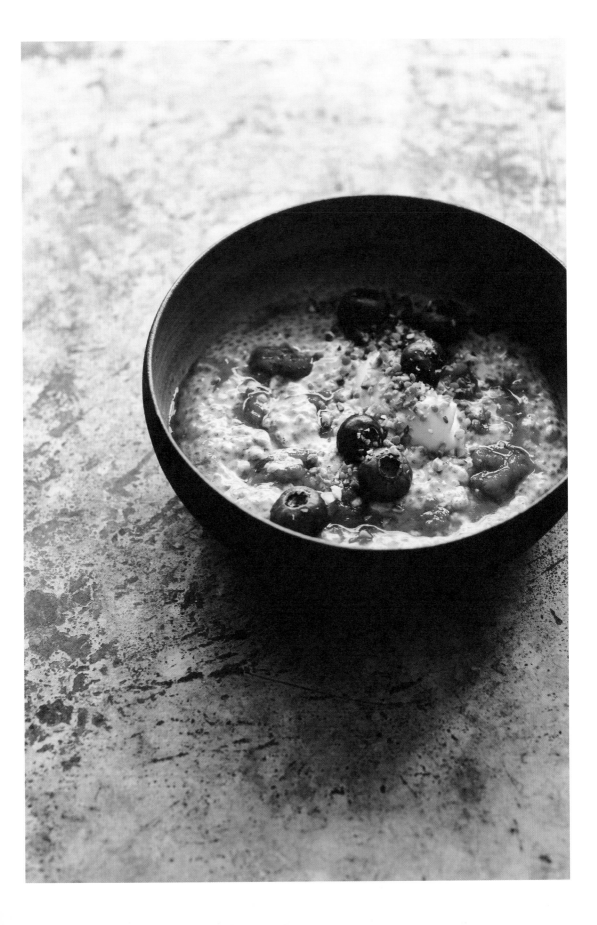

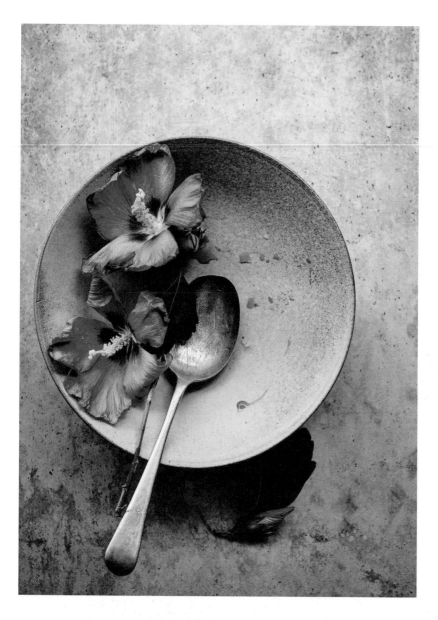

A BALANCED ROOT CHAKRA PLAYS A SIGNIFICANT PART IN YOUR OVERALL HEALTH. WHEN IT'S IN BALANCE, WITH NO BLOCKAGES, YOU'RE LIKELY TO FEEL HEALTHY, STABLE, RELAXED, TRUSTING, SECURE AND PROSPEROUS. YOU WILL HAVE AN ABUNDANCE OF ENERGY AS WELL AS THE ABILITY TO THINK ABUNDANTLY IN ALL AREAS OF LIFE. FEELINGS OF CENTEREDNESS, CALM AND ORGANIZATION WILL ABOUND. PEOPLE MAY DESCRIBE YOU AS HAVING A LOT OF COMMON SENSE AND YOU'LL FEEL AT EASE WITH YOURSELF – MENTALLY AND PHYSICALLY.

AN OUT-OF-BALANCE ROOT CHAKRA MAY INDUCE A LACK OF ABILITY TO FOCUS OR STAY MOTIVATED AS WELL AS VULNERABILITY, PARANOIA, AGGRESSION, A QUICK TEMPER, INSECURITY, INABILITY TO RELAX, AND ANXIETY.

In order to create the life you want to live, you need to find your centre and get grounded. Being grounded creates the platform on which you feel secure, gives you a sense of belonging, and connects you to the physical world. When grounded, you will find yourself confident, open to new things, and taking measures towards your goals and dreams.

But when life gives you lemons, your security and sense of belonging are disrupted and life can feel unstable. You may dig your heels in and revert to your routines in order to consolidate. While routines are essential and offer many benefits, life tends to become stagnant if you allow it to.

Staying in survival mode closes us off to the vibrant, unexpected excitement life has to offer, and for that reason, I included this smoothie recipe using the beautiful hibiscus flower. Not only is it gorgeous to look at, it's not an ingredient you might have thought to include in your smoothie. It offers a deep crimson colour to any liquid and its tart flavour is reminiscent of pomegranate or cranberry, and you may be surprised by its lemon notes and delicate robustness. Substitute for a rich berry-flavoured tea bag or fruit powders such as acai, cherry or pomegranate if you need to.

COCONUT DREAM HIBISCUS & BERRY SMOOTHIE (v)

SERVES 2

1½ teaspoons hibiscus powder, or 2 hibiscus flower tea bags
400ml (14fl oz/1¾ cups) can full-fat coconut milk
125g (4½oz/1 cup) frozen raspberries
1 ripe banana
1 teaspoon lucuma powder (optional)
6–8 ice cubes (optional)

If you are using the hibiscus flower tea bags, steep them in 300ml (1¼ cups) of boiling water. Leave the tea bags in the boiling water and allow to cool completely. You may want to do this the night before or before you leave the house in the morning.

To make the smoothie, blend all the ingredients in a blender for 2–3 minutes. Pour into 2 glasses and enjoy.

This salad makes a great dinner-party starter, as it is so colourful and vibrant to look at, or a simple salad you can make for lunch. If you're short on time then you can always thinly slice the beetroot using a mandolin instead of roasting them. A versatile salad that hits the spot every time!

FENNEL, BEETROOT, BALSAMIC & ORANGE SALAD
with whipped feta

SERVES 2

2 beetroot (beets), red or golden
2 tablespoons extra virgin olive oil, plus a drizzle for cooking the beetroot, and extra to serve, if wished
1 large fennel bulb (fronds reserved)
2 teaspoons freshly squeezed orange juice
2 teaspoons freshly squeezed lemon juice
1 red chicory (endive), leaves trimmed, removed and washed
a handful of rocket (arugula) leaves
2 oranges, peeled and segmented
1 teaspoon balsamic glaze
sea salt and cracked black pepper

FOR THE FETA
WHIPPED RICOTTA
60g (2oz/½ cup) diced feta cheese
60g (2oz/¼ cup) ricotta
2 teaspoons extra virgin olive oil

Preheat the oven to 180°C/350°F/Gas 4.

Rinse and scrub the beetroot under cold water. Place in a large bowl and toss with a drizzle of olive oil and a little salt and pepper. Wrap each beetroot in kitchen foil and place on a large baking sheet. Roast the beetroot for 1 hour (or longer, depending on the size), or until the beetroot can be easily pierced all the way through with a sharp knife. Once the beetroot are cooked through, set aside on a plate (keep them wrapped in foil) until they are cool enough to handle. Trim the ends, peel, and cut into segments. Set aside.

Trim the top and bottom of the fennel bulb and slice the bulb in half lengthways. Remove the core of the fennel bulb with a sharp knife, and slice or mandolin each cored half crossways into thin slices, roughly 2mm (⅛in) thick.

Place the sliced fennel in a mixing bowl. Add the olive oil, orange and lemon juice, and toss gently to combine. Season to taste and set aside.

For the feta whipped ricotta, combine the feta, ricotta, olive oil and salt and pepper to taste in the bowl of a mini food processor. Pulse until very smooth. Transfer to a small bowl and set aside.

To serve, distribute the chicory and rocket leaves onto 2 plates, then layer with the fennel mixture, orange segments, beetroot and the balsamic glaze. Serve with a dollop of the feta whipped ricotta on the side. Drizzle lightly with extra virgin olive oil if desired.

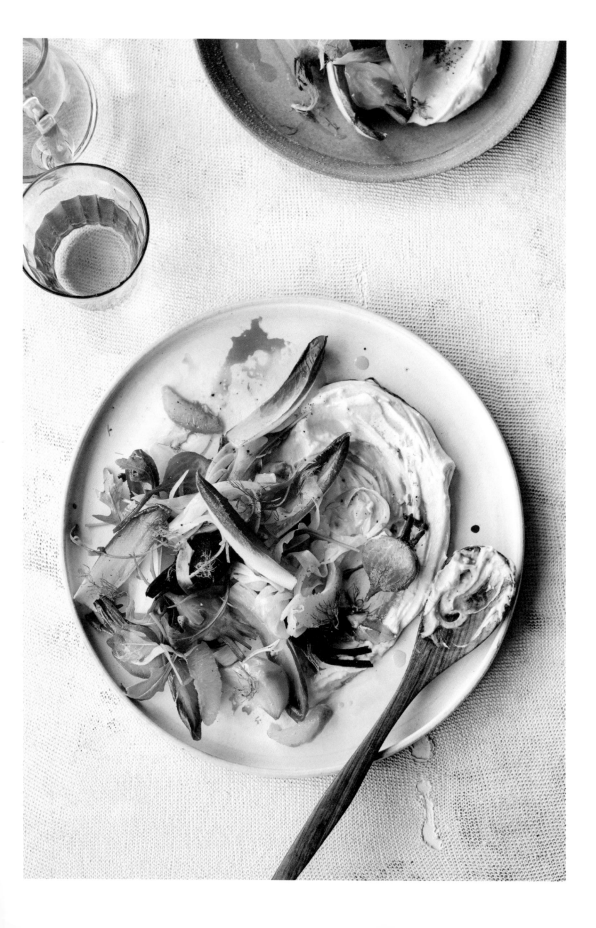

This is the kind of bowl food I love to linger over. A true grounding root chakra experience, where time seems to stop and transport you to a space where you can achieve inner connection.

If you're a traditionalist, you can substitute the Parmesan back into this pesto recipe, or if you're up for trying the vegan version, I bet you won't even miss the cheese.

THRIVE GRATITUDE BOWL
with apple & beetroot sauerkraut (v)

SERVES 2

FOR THE VEGAN
PESTO QUINOA

90g (3¼oz) basil, stalks and
  leaves included
3 tablespoons nutritional
  yeast flakes
70g (2½oz/heaped ½ cup) pine
  nuts/kernels
1 teaspoon sea salt
150ml (5fl oz/⅔ cup) extra virgin
  olive oil, plus more if needed
  and 50ml (3½ tablespoons)
  for storage
60g (2oz/⅓ cup) quinoa, washed

FOR THE APPLE &
BEETROOT SAUERKRAUT

600g (1lb 5oz) red cabbage,
  finely shredded using a
  mandolin
1 tablespoon sea salt
1 medium–large beetroot (beet),
  peeled and grated
2 eating apples, cored and grated
2 star anise

Begin my making the sauerkraut and don't worry if you haven't made this in advance. I'll show you how to make the fuller version here, but if you want a quick and easy version for this salad today, see the tip over the page.

Using your hands, massage the cabbage and salt together in a large mixing bowl for 2 minutes. As you squeeze and mix the cabbage you should start to notice the moisture coming out of it. Add the grated beetroot and apple, and the star anise and mix to combine. Place the cabbage mixture into a glass jar or the next best thing would be a glass Tupperware with an airtight lid. If you don't have glass, then a plastic Tupperware will do too. Push the mixture firmly down into your jar or Tupperware, removing any gaps. Add enough water to the container to cover the top of the cabbage by 2cm (¾in).

Taking a piece of muslin, cheesecloth or clean kitchen towel, secure the cloth around the outside of the container with an elastic band, place the sauerkraut on a tray and set aside in a cool, dark place overnight to start the fermenting process. Leave the container on the tray at room temperature for 3–5 days, topping up with water as necessary to ensure the sauerkraut is always covered. You will know your sauerkraut is ready when bubbles start to appear on the surface. Once the sauerkraut is ready, remove the cloth and top with 2cm (¾in) of water again before refrigerating. The sauerkraut will keep for up to 1 month in the fridge.

INGREDIENTS & METHOD CONTINUE...

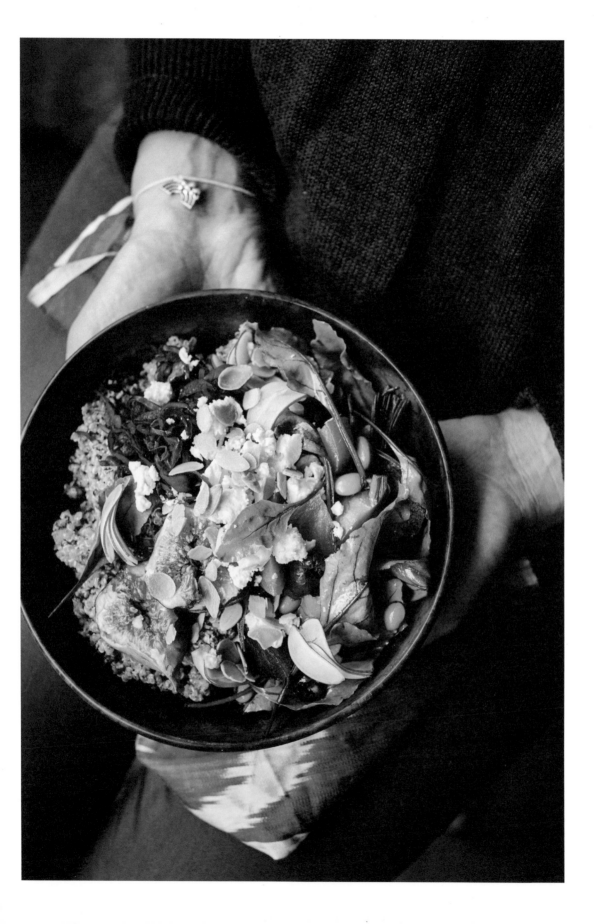

CONTINUED...

FOR THE DRESSING
2 tablespoons olive oil
1 tablespoon balsamic vinegar
1 tablespoon maple syrup
sea salt and cracked black pepper

FOR THE SALAD
2–3 store-bought cooked
 beetroots (beets)
3 radishes, thinly sliced into rounds
40g (1½oz/⅓ cup) edamame
 beans
1 tablespoon pitted black olives,
 roughly chopped
1 handful baby red chard or
 spinach leaves

TO SERVE
2 fresh figs
toasted almonds, roughly chopped
goat's cheese or feta cheese
 (optional, if vegan)

To make the pesto, put the basil, yeast, pine nuts, salt and olive oil in a food processor and blend until smooth. Add a little more oil to reach your desired consistency and taste for seasoning. Remove from the food processor and store in a glass jar or tall Tupperware container. Top with the 50ml (3½ tablespoons) olive oil. The olive oil acts as a preservative to prevent your pesto from spoiling. Always make sure the pesto jar has a layer of olive oil and your pesto will last for weeks!

To cook the quinoa, put the quinoa in a small saucepan, add enough cold water to cover by 1cm (½in), then bring to the boil and cook for 10–12 minutes, or until all the water has evaporated. Quickly remove from the heat and place a clean kitchen towel over the saucepan and secure a lid tightly over the tea towel creating a seal. Set aside and allow the quinoa to cool and become light and fluffy as the moisture is absorbed by the tea towel.

Meanwhile, make the salad dressing by mixing all the ingredients together and seasoning with salt and pepper.

To make the salad, cut the beetroot into wedges. Add to a mixing bowl with the sliced radishes, edamame beans and black olives. Add the baby chard or spinach leaves and toss to combine. Set aside.

Place the cooked quinoa into a mixing bowl and add as much or as little of the pesto as you desire to give the quinoa a lovely green colour.

To serve, place the salad into bowls of your choice, add some pesto quinoa and the apple and beetroot sauerkraut. Tear each fig between your fingers and place flesh over the top of each bowl, sprinkle with toasted almonds and goat's or feta cheese, if desired.

QUICK TIP
For a quick version of the apple and beetroot sauerkraut, you can take a store-bought jar of plain sauerkraut, add some grated beetroot and apple, plus 1 tablespoon grated ginger for flavour. Mix to combine and you have ready-to-use, gorgeously colourful and flavoursome sauerkraut in less than 5 minutes!

52

Two of the best ways to balance your root chakra are to eat mindfully and include comfort foods like root vegetables into your day-to-day diet. By eating as many vegetables as possible that have been grown in the earth, you bring a grounding frequency into your body, which can help alleviate any out-of-balance feelings. This lasagne can be a great place to start. I have used thinly cut celeriac slices instead of pasta sheets here and created an earthy flavoured tomato sauce with green lentils and garam masala.

Omit the Parmesan for a vegan version or try topping with the nut cheese from the blackberry soup recipe on page 148.

CELERIAC 'PASTA' LASAGNA

SERVES 2

FOR THE TOMATO SAUCE

1 tablespoon extra virgin olive oil, plus extra to drizzle
3 celery sticks, finely diced
2 tablespoons tomato purée (paste)
1 x 400g (14oz) can green lentils
1 x 400g (14oz) can chopped tomatoes
½ teaspoon garam masala
1 teaspoon sea salt
1 tablespoon finely chopped flat-leaf parsley leaves

TO ASSEMBLE

¼ large celeriac (celery root), peeled and cut into long thin sheets
40g (1½oz/½ cup) grated Parmesan cheese
½ large aubergine (eggplant), cut into long thin sheets
1 courgette (zucchini), cut into thin strips using a peeler

Begin by making the tomato sauce. Place a non-stick saucepan over a medium heat, add the olive oil and celery and sauté for 2–3 minutes or until soft and translucent. Add the tomato purée and 50ml (3½ tablespoons) water and stir to combine. Now add the can of lentils including the juices and the can of chopped tomatoes. Add the garam masala and stir to combine. Bring to a light simmer and cover with a lid. Simmer for 10 minutes. Remove from the heat and add the sea salt and parsley.

Preheat the oven to 180°C/350°F/Gas 4. To assemble the lasagna, spread a thin layer of tomato sauce in the bottom of a 28 x 18cm (11¼ x 7in) baking dish. Place a layer of celeriac sheets over the top of the sauce. Add another layer of sauce and a sprinkle of Parmesan. Now place a layer of aubergine and continue layering the tomato sauce, Parmesan, celeriac and aubergine until all the tomato sauce has been used, but making sure you save some Parmesan for the top. For the final layer, lattice the courgette ribbons over the top of the lasagne. Drizzle with olive oil, then sprinkle a final layer of Parmesan over the courgette lattice.

Cover the dish with kitchen foil and bake for 45 minutes. Remove the foil and bake for a further 10–15 minutes, or until the lasagna is a little crispy and the vegetable layers are cooked through. Remove from the oven and allow to sit for 15 minutes before serving.

If there is one recipe I crave, then it is this one. It's a real showstopper served to guests who may want to join you on the plan for a night.

This is best eaten directly after baking, but it is also good to have in the house for quick and easy post-yoga fuel.

HARVEST HASSELBACKS

with sage-wrapped baby carrots, spiced maple juices, & chunky walnut & date yoghurt

SERVES 2

2 small–medium beetroots (beets), trimmed and peeled
2 small sweet potatoes
2 parsnips, trimmed and peeled
1 courgette (zucchini)
20g (⅔oz/1½ tablespoons) unsalted butter, melted
10g (⅓oz/scant ¼ cup) grated Parmesan cheese
15g (½oz/¼ cup) fresh breadcrumbs
sea salt and cracked black pepper
2 handfuls rocket (arugula) leaves, to serve

FOR THE SAGE CARROTS

500g (1lb 2oz, about 16) mixed heirloom baby carrots or normal baby carrots, trimmed and peeled
About 16 sage leaves
About 16 whole cloves
2 bay leaves
4 strips orange peel, plus freshly squeezed juice of 1 orange
2 tablespoons maple syrup
2 tablespoons extra virgin olive oil, plus extra for greasing

FOR THE WALNUT & DATE YOGHURT

65g (2¼oz/¼ cup) full-fat, natural Greek yoghurt
35g (1¼oz/⅓ cup) dates, pitted and roughly chopped
25g (1oz/¼ cup) walnuts, toasted and roughly chopped
1 tablespoon extra virgin olive oil

Preheat the oven to 200°C/400°F/Gas 6. Line a roasting tray with baking paper.

At 3–6mm (⅛–¼in) intervals, cut very thin slices into each of the beetroots, sweet potatoes, parsnips and courgette, making sure to cut deep but not all the way through each vegetable so that they hold together at the bottom. Place in the roasting tray, drizzle over half of the melted butter and season with salt and pepper. Roast in the preheated oven for 1 hour, then remove from oven. Combine the cheese and breadcrumbs and sprinkle it over the vegetables. Drizzle with the remaining butter and return to the oven to roast for a further 10 minutes or until golden.

While the hasselbacks are in the oven, make the carrots. Wrap each carrot in a sage leaf, then secure in place by pressing a whole clove into the overlap of the sage leaf and carrot. Place the wrapped carrots into a lightly greased roasting tray large enough for all the carrots to fit in a single layer. Add the bay leaves, orange peel and orange juice. Drizzle with the olive oil and maple syrup and sprinkle with salt and pepper. Add 120ml (4fl oz/½ cup) water and cover the roasting tray with kitchen foil. Roast for 20 minutes, then remove the foil and continue to cook for another 10–20 minutes or until the carrots are cooked through and firm. Remove the carrots from the oven and cover with foil to keep warm.

To make the chunky walnut & date yoghurt, loosen the yoghurt by giving it a stir, then add the dates, walnuts and the olive oil and stir to combine. Keep cool until ready to serve.

To serve, remove the hasselbacks from the oven and cut the courgette in half. Place a handful of rocket and half a courgette onto each serving plate. Divide the hasselbacks and carrots between the plates and serve with a dollop of the chunky walnut and date yoghurt.

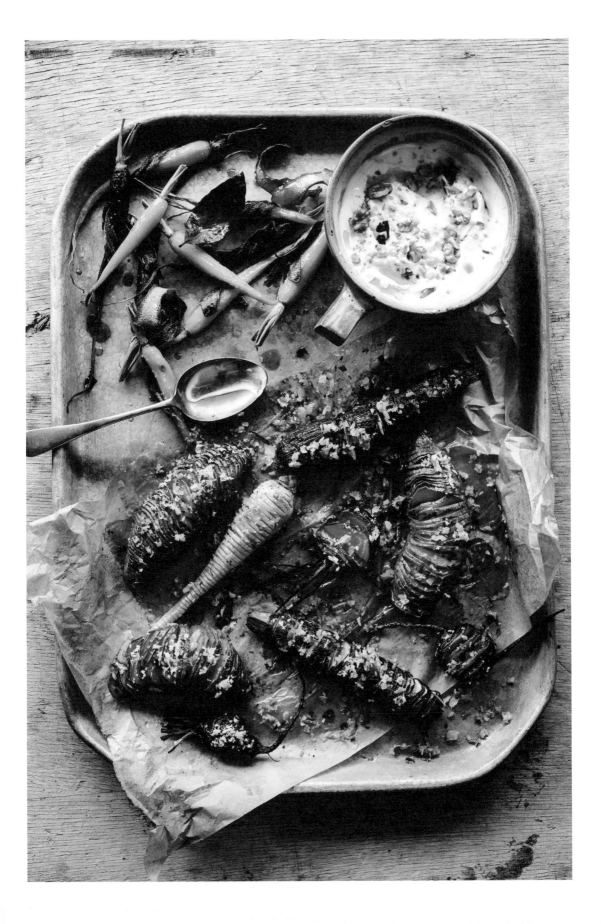

SACRAL CHAKRA
honour

Key foods for the sacral chakra:
ORANGE FOOD: papaya, mango, orange, carrot,
squash, sweet potato, apricot
FOOD FOR DIGESTIVE HEALTH: fermented foods,
such as miso, tempeh, kimchi, sauerkraut, kefir,
kombucha, tamari, full-fat live yoghurt etc.
FOOD FOR REPRODUCTIVE HEALTH:
maca root powder, kelp
Enjoy sourdough bread and avoid refined sugars,
protein-rich foods and hard-to-digest foods

If papaya is unavailable substitute with mango, nectarine or peach to make the smoothie bowl mixture. In the cooler months, when a smoothie bowl may not suit, make a smoothie instead using ingredients at room temperature.

Papayas are freshest when at high season in early summer, but owing to their commercial cultivation they can be found all year round. The trick is to choose a ripe papaya with a deep yellow or orange skin and similar colour flesh. Of course you certainly don't have to serve your smoothie bowl inside a side of papaya: be creative and use other ripe fruits such as half a melon or simply serve in a cute breakfast bowl.

PAPAYA & RASPBERRY SMOOTHIE BOWL
with passion fruit curd (v)

SERVES 2

FOR THE SMOOTHIE BOWL

1 ripe papaya
freshly squeezed juice of ½ lemon
2 ripe bananas, sliced into 2cm (¾in) slices and frozen
½ avocado, peeled, stoned and diced into 2cm (¾in) pieces and frozen
120g (4¼oz/1 cup) frozen raspberries
4 tablespoons beetroot (beet) juice
2 tablespoons coconut butter (optional)
2 tablespoons vanilla vegan protein powder

FOR THE PASSION FRUIT CURD

3 ripe passion fruits
1 tablespoon freshly squeezed lemon juice
1 tablespoon coconut butter

FOR THE TOPPINGS

raspberries
kiwi fruit, cut in half and into jagged edges
toasted coconut flakes
bee pollen (optional, if vegan)

Begin by making the passion fruit curd. Halve each passion fruit and remove the pulp and seeds using a teaspoon. Put the pulp in a small saucepan, then add the lemon juice and coconut butter and whisk over a low heat until the coconut butter has been incorporated. Transfer the curd to a glass jar and place in the fridge while you begin making the smoothie bowl mixture.

Slice the papaya in half lengthways. Remove all the seeds using a dessertspoon and discard. Then, using the same dessertspoon, carefully remove a 5mm (¼in) thick layer of the ripe flesh from each papaya half and place in a blender or food processor. Set the papaya halves aside.

Add the remaining smoothie-bowl ingredients to your blender and blend on high speed until smooth. You may need to use the blender paddle or a silicone spatula to make sure all the ingredients are incorporated and smooth.

Spoon the smoothie bowl contents into the scooped-out papaya, then top with your desired toppings and the passion fruit curd. Enjoy, making sure you spoon out the rest of the papaya flesh along the way.

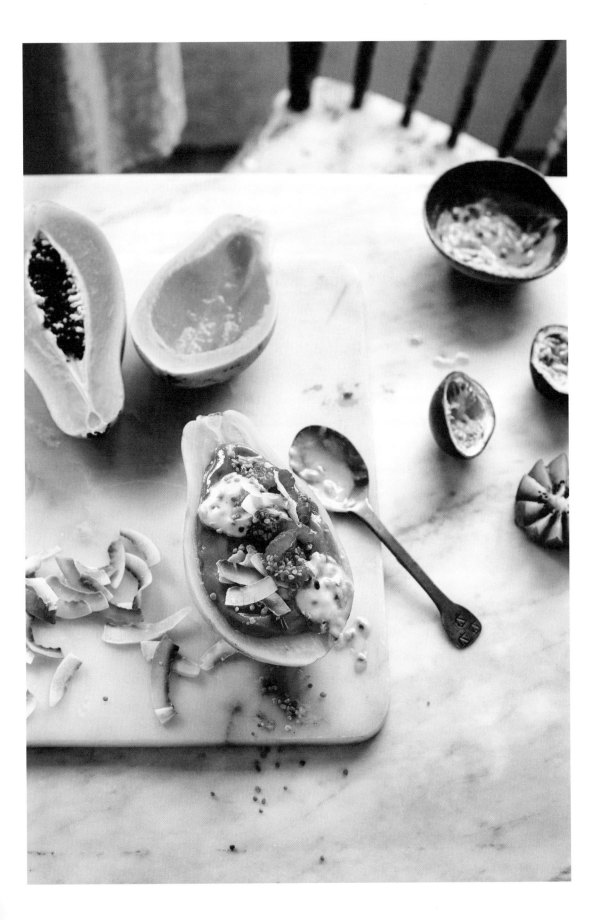

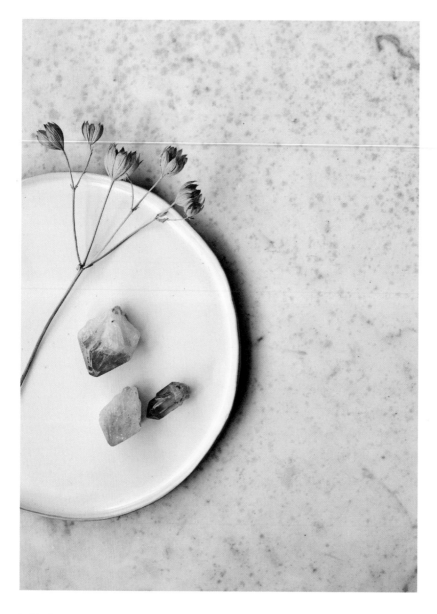

I GIVE MYSELF PERMISSION TO ENJOY LIFE
AND BE CREATIVE TODAY.

My dad, a man who loves his porridge, milky and sweet but plain, will kick me for saying this, but I often find oats cooked in the simplest porridge form a little too boring. For me, oats need bringing to life with exciting ingredients like when they are baked into granola with loads of whole nuts, or used to combine courgette, feta and olives in the savoury flapjack from my original *The Yoga Kitchen* book.

Far from the cold, Oxford mornings from his upbringing, I grew up with Australian sunshine brightening our kitchen table and the quickest and easiest way to make breakfast oats seem sexy was to whip a flavourful punch of creamy yoghurt through them and then add grated apple and some nuts.

Although I haven't instructed you to soak the oats overnight, you certainly can, as the oats will soften to create an even creamier texture. If you decide to make the oats the night before, follow the instructions up until the point before you add the pomegranate seeds and pistachios. Cover the oats overnight and, in the morning, whip through the pomegranate seeds and pistachios and then serve and garnish.

COCONUT & MANGO YOGHURT BREAKFAST BIRCHER (v)

SERVES 2

FOR THE BIRCHER

85g (3oz/⅓ cup) coconut yoghurt
80g (2¾oz) mango, puréed
1 eating apple, grated
80g (2¾oz/¾ cup) rolled oats
1 tablespoon freshly squeezed
  lemon juice
2 tablespoons pomegranate seeds
1 tablespoon raw pistachios,
  roughly chopped

TO GARNISH (OPTIONAL)

coconut flakes
buckwheat groats
pomegranate seeds
raw pistachios, roughly chopped

Place the yoghurt and puréed mango in a mixing bowl. Stir so the mango and yoghurt are completely incorporated. Add the grated apple, rolled oats and lemon juice. Stir to combine, then fold through the pomegranate seeds and chopped pistachios.

The bircher will be a gorgeous, light orange colour. Taste the bircher and adjust for sweetness and flavour. You may like to add a little extra lemon juice.

Serve the bircher in breakfast bowls topped with coconut flakes, buckwheat groats plus extra pistachios and pomegranate seeds, if you wish. Enjoy it immediately or keep it in the fridge for 3–5 days.

I am a big believer in choosing the most nutrient-dense foods to include in your diet, so while some of you may roll your eyes at the idea of spirulina being whipped through your yoghurt, be grateful someone is looking out for you, making sure you get your dose of greens with every meal!

SPICED MAPLE, PECAN & ORANGE GRANOLA
with fresh berry salad & redemption yoghurt (v)

SERVES 2–4

40g (1½oz/¼ cup) buckwheat groats
100g (3½oz/1 cup) rolled oats
90g (3¼oz/¾ cup) pecans
40g dried (1½oz/⅓ cup) cranberries
2 tablespoons pumpkin seeds
1½ tablespoons flaxseeds
½ tablespoon ground cinnamon
1 teaspoon ground allspice
a pinch of sea salt
zest of 1 orange
½ teaspoon vanilla extract
4½ tablespoons maple syrup
2½ tablespoons extra virgin olive oil

FOR THE BERRY SALAD

50g (1¾oz/⅓ cup) raspberries
50g (1¾oz/⅓ cup) blueberries
50g (1¾oz/½ cup) strawberries, trimmed and cut into quarters

FOR THE REDEMPTION YOGHURT

2 teaspoons maple syrup
½ teaspoon spirulina powder
6 tablespoons full-fat, natural yoghurt (vegan if necessary)

To make the granola, preheat the oven to 160°C/315°F/Gas 2–3 and line a baking sheet with baking paper. Now add all the ingredients to a large mixing bowl and stir to completely combine, coating all the dry ingredients in the maple syrup and olive oil.

Spread the granola mixture over the baking sheet and bake for 50–60 minutes until golden in colour and when you lift the edge of the baking paper up at the corner the granola can be lifted in clumps and looks golden on the underside. Allow to cool completely on the sheet before touching – this will keep the characteristic clumps from breaking apart.

To make the berry salad, combine all the berries in a small bowl.

To make the redemption yoghurt, place the maple syrup and spirulina powder in a small bowl and whisk until the spirulina dissolves, making sure there are no lumps of spirulina. Add the yoghurt and whisk to combine.

To serve, divide the granola and berry salad between 2 breakfast bowls and add the yoghurt. Serve immediately.

The granola can be kept in an airtight jar or container for 3–6 months.

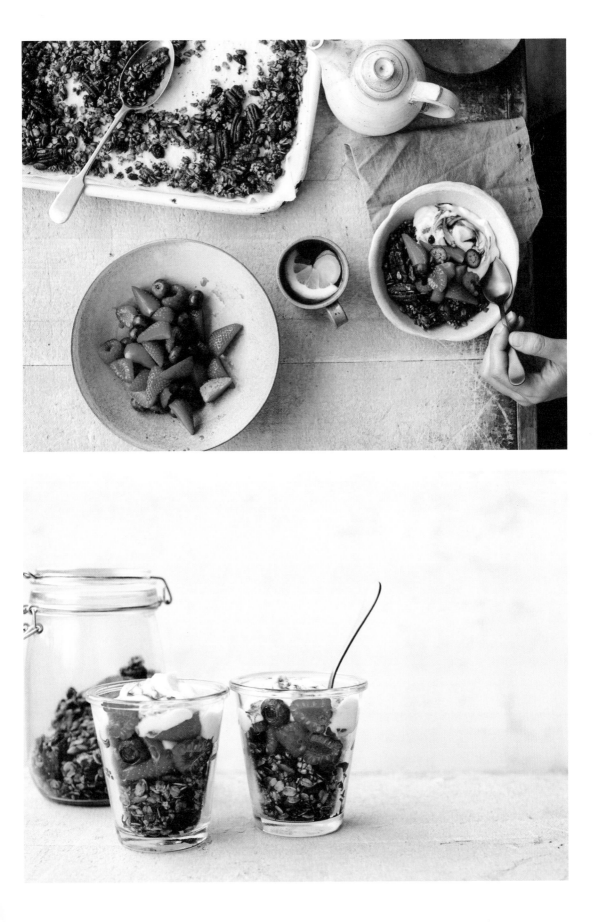

If you haven't begun to see the trend already, I am going to give it away here; my favourite meals of the day are breakfast and dessert and in a book where there are no desserts, I just had to sneak in a few indulgent breakfasts. This is certainly one of them.

SPELT PANCAKES
served with caramelized bananas & sweet chestnut sauce (v)

SERVES 2

160g (5¾oz/scant 1¼ cups) spelt flour (or buckwheat flour if a gluten-free flour is preferred)
1 teaspoon baking powder
½ teaspoon bicarbonate of soda (baking soda)
1 tablespoon coconut sugar
1 tablespoon ground flaxseed
½ teaspoon ground cinnamon
a pinch of salt
1 teaspoon fresh lemon juice
1 teaspoon vanilla extract
1 tablespoon olive oil, plus extra for greasing
130ml (4½fl oz/generous ½ cup) oat milk, or milk of your choice
2 bananas, mashed

FOR THE CHESTNUT SAUCE

90g (3¼oz/scant 1 cup) cooked chestnuts
2 tablespoons maple syrup
1 teaspoon vanilla extract
a pinch of sea salt

FOR THE CARAMELIZED BANANAS

2 tablespoons maple syrup
2 tablespoons coconut sugar
1 teaspoon coconut oil
2 ripe bananas, peeled and cut lengthways

TO SERVE

kefir, or yoghurt of your choice
blueberries (optional)
macadamia nuts, walnuts or any nut of your choice (optional)

To make the pancake batter, put the flour, baking powder, bicarbonate of soda, coconut sugar, ground flaxseed, cinnamon and salt into a mixing bowl. Stir to combine, then add all the wet ingredients to the bowl and stir to completely combine. Set aside for 5 minutes while you make the sweet chestnut sauce.

In a small food processor or blender, add the chestnuts, maple syrup, 100ml (3½fl oz/scant ½ cup) water, vanilla and sea salt. Blend on high speed for 1–2 minutes until a smooth sauce is formed. Taste and add a little extra maple syrup if desired. If you would like your sauce a little runnier, add some more water too. Set the sauce aside and start making the pancakes.

Place a non-stick frying pan over a medium–high heat. While waiting for the pan to heat, brush with a little olive oil and then lower the heat to medium. Using a soup ladle, spoon half a ladle of batter into the frying pan and gently spread to create a round pancake. Once there are bubbles on top of the pancake and its edges have started to look a little cooked, flip the pancake over and cook for a further minute or so. Remove the pancake from the pan and place on a warmed plate. Repeat this process to use all the remaining batter to make 6 pancakes in total.

While the pancakes are being made, place another non-stick frying pan over a medium heat for the caramelized bananas. Add the maple syrup, coconut sugar and oil, stir, then add the banana, cut faces down, into the syrup. Allow the banana and syrup to bubble for a few minutes. Remove from the heat.

To serve, place a stack of 3 pancakes in the middle of a plate, drizzle with some chestnut sauce, then spoon a dollop of yoghurt over the top. Gently remove the caramelized bananas from the pan, crisscross them over the yoghurt and drizzle with any caramel from the pan. Drizzle with a little more chestnut sauce, and add some blueberries and chopped macadamia nuts or walnuts, if desired. Enjoy while still warm.

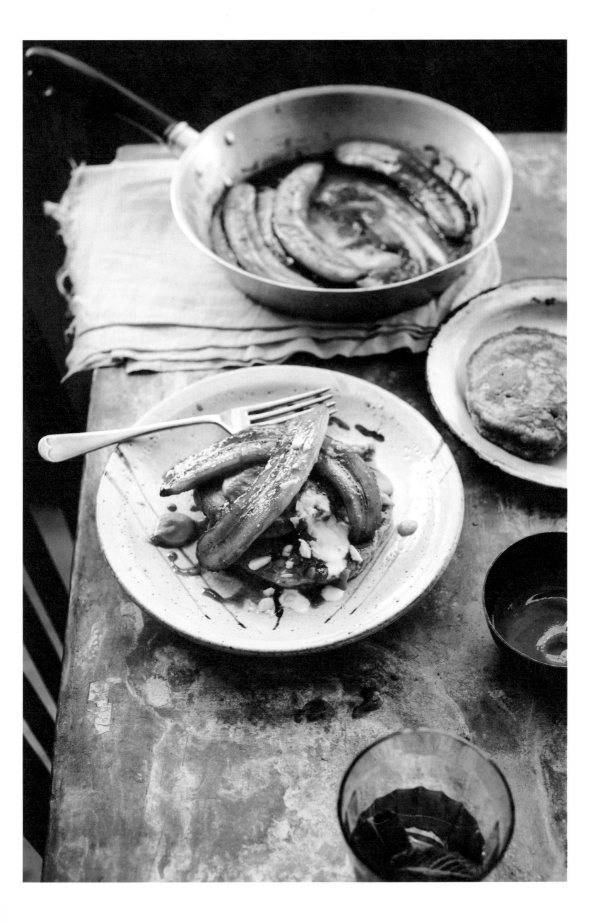

You can almost taste the sunshine in every juice-laden mouthful of summer's mangoes in this recipe. Inspired by the lush, fresh flavours of my home, Australia, this salad shows how you can transform raw ingredients into a light and zesty meal that delivers an abundance of vitality with every bite.

There is no need for a salad dressing here, as the coconut and mango are naturally wet and juicy anyway. The simplest sprinkle of lime zest and chilli flakes is all it needs to bring this salad together.

MANGO, MINT, COCONUT & CHILLI SALAD (v)

SERVES 2

flesh of 1 young coconut
2 mangoes, peeled, pitted and flesh chopped into thin slices
a small handful of mint leaves
freshly squeezed juice of 1 lime
1 tablespoon apple cider vinegar
½ teaspoon dried chilli (hot pepper) flakes
½ teaspoon finely grated lime zest
toasted cashews, to serve
sea salt flakes, to serve

Wash the coconut flesh and discard any husk, then break the flesh up into 2.5cm (1in) pieces using your hands.

Place the coconut, mangoes, mint, lime juice, vinegar, chilli flakes and lime zest in a bowl and toss to combine.

Divide into individual bowls and top with toasted cashews and sea salt to serve.

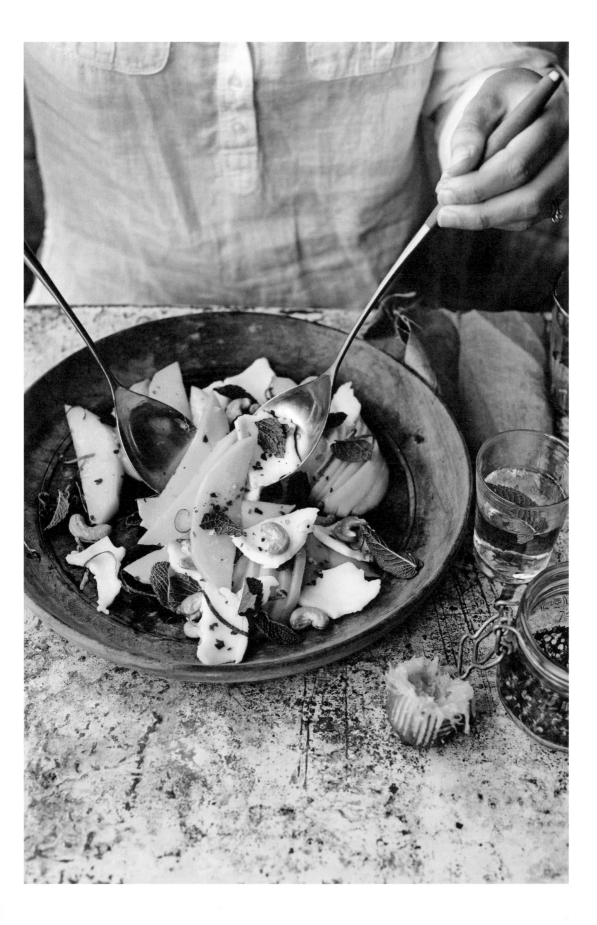

I love this kind of food – a real sensory overload! Fresh, crisp ingredients that are clean on their own but mouthwateringly moreish once dressed up with vibrant flavours.

You can substitute the peanut butter for cashew butter if you like. And if I were you, I would make a double batch of this satay sauce, because once its gone, you'll wish you had more.

TEMPEH SATAY SKEWERS
with carrot, mooli & edamame slaw (v)

SERVES 4

FOR THE SLAW

1 mooli (white radish/daikon) – or an additional 2 carrots
2–3 large carrots
150g (5½oz/1¼ cups) edamame beans
8 pink radishes, thinly sliced
4 spring onions (scallions), trimmed and thinly sliced
125g (4½oz/heaped 2 cups) bean sprouts, washed
20g (⅔oz/1 cup) coriander (cilantro) leaves, roughly chopped
20g (⅔oz/1 cup) mint leaves, roughly chopped

FOR THE DRESSING

5 tablespoons sweet chilli sauce
5 tablespoons toasted sesame oil
3 tablespoons tamari sauce
1 tablespoon rice wine vinegar
freshly squeezed juice of 2 limes
1 teaspoon white and/or black sesame seeds

FOR THE SATAY

5 tablespoons smooth peanut butter
1 teaspoon Thai red curry paste
2 tablespoons rice wine vinegar
2 tablespoons tamari sauce
1 tablespoon tamarind paste
600g (1lb 5oz) tempeh or firm tofu, cut into thick batons
1 tablespoon extra virgin olive oil

To make the slaw, peel the mooli and carrots, trim the tops and bases and grate them using a large grater, or for speed and ease pass them through the grater blade of your food processor. Now, place the grated carrot and mooli into ice-cold water while you prepare the rest of the slaw and its dressing.

To make the dressing, put all the ingredients in a small bowl and whisk to combine.

In a large bowl combine the edamame beans, radishes, spring onions and bean sprouts. Drain and dry the carrots and mooli, then add them to the rest of the salad ingredients. Now add the herbs and dressing and toss to combine. Once the salad is coated in the dressing, set aside in the fridge while you make the almond satay and tempeh skewers.

To make the satay, put the peanut butter, Thai red curry paste, vinegar, tamari, tamarind paste and 5 tablespoons water into a bowl and stir until smooth and well combined.

Preheat a griddle (char-grill) pan over a high heat. Thread the tempeh onto 8 metal skewers and brush with half the satay. Brush the griddle with olive oil and cook the skewers, turning regularly, for 6–8 minutes or until golden and charred.

To serve, place a portion of slaw onto each plate and then top with 2 skewers. Drizzle the remaining satay sauce over the plates and serve.

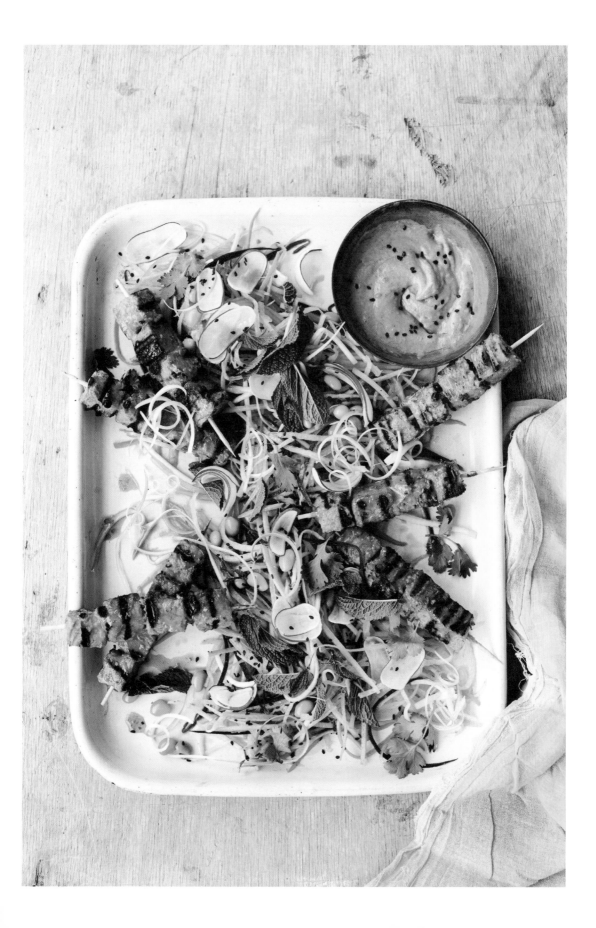

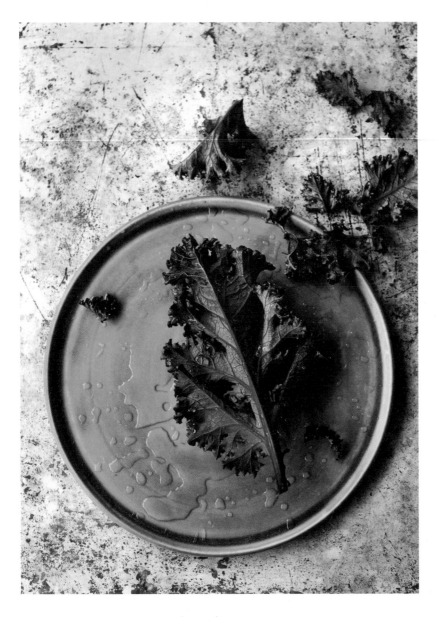

AT TIMES WHEN I FEEL A LITTLE 'STUCK' OR THAT LIFE IS OUT
OF BALANCE, I LIKE TO GET OUT MY NOTEPAD AND WRITE AT
THE TOP OF THE PAGE "I AM LOOKING FORWARD TO FEELING…"
AND THEN I BEGIN TO LIST ALL THE THINGS THAT I AM HOPING
AND WISHING FOR AND THAT I MAY NOT BE EXPERIENCING AT
THE TIME. JUST THIS PROCESS HELPS ME TO FIGURE OUT HOW
I MIGHT ATTAIN SOME OF THE FEELINGS THAT SEEM TO BE
MISSING, AND TO SEE HOW I CAN ADJUST SO THAT I AM OPEN
TO FOSTERING THEM IN MY LIFE. TRY IT NEXT TIME YOU ARE
FEELING LIKE LIFE NEEDS A LITTLE MORE SPICE OR YOU JUST
DON'T SEEM TO BE FEELING THE WAY YOU WANT TO ON A
DAILY BASIS.

The sacral chakra is the home of your sexuality, emotions and creativity, guiding you to see beyond the mundane to embrace your dreams and desires. It also governs your ability to initiate, nurture and maintain healthy interpersonal relationships.

The first sign that your sacral chakra is out of balance is a general lack of vitality. You may find yourself struggling with work with a consistent feeling that life is nothing more than a daily grind. Your ability to spontaneously feel joy or to be playful has a way of vanishing when the sacral chakra is weakened, closed or imbalanced.

People whose sacral chakra is in balance are usually wonderful to be around. They are open to life and to everything happening around them and they convey an inner joy and radiance that is contagious.

SQUASH & LENTIL KORMA
with coriander & mint (v)

SERVES 2

500g (1lb 2 oz) butternut squash, peeled, deseeded and cut into 2cm (¾in) chunks
100g (3½oz/scant ½ cup) store-bought korma curry paste
1 x 400ml (14fl oz) can full-fat coconut milk
200g (7oz/1½ cups) drained and rinsed canned lentils
200g (7oz/1½ cups) drained and rinsed canned chickpeas (garbanzo beans)
75g (2½oz) curly kale, stalk removed and roughly chopped
freshly squeezed juice of 1 lime
sea salt

TO SERVE

flaked (slivered) almonds, toasted
mint leaves
coriander (cilantro) leaves

Place the squash chunks, curry paste and coconut milk into a wide heavy-based saucepan over a low–medium heat. Stir to combine, dissolving the curry paste into the coconut milk. Cover and simmer for 20 minutes. Stir in the lentils and chickpeas and bring back to a light simmer, then cook until the squash is tender and cooked through.

Remove the pan from the heat. Add the kale, stir through and allow it to wilt from the heat of the korma juices. Stir through the lime juice, season to taste, and serve. Sprinkle each plate with toasted almonds, plus a few mint and coriander leaves.

I am a big fan of the one-pan style of cooking, not only because of its simplicity and lack of cooking attention that it needs, but also because it means there is only a chopping board, knife and tray to wash up afterwards.

But more than anything, one-pan tray bakes pack a flavourful punch as the juices of each ingredient begin to blend with each other, which just helps to intensify the aromatic and taste-bud experience.

In this tray bake, the juices from the tomatoes gorgeously melt into the juices from the kalamata olives, giving the halloumi an unexpected sauce, while the kale becomes crisp and crunchy to contrast the soft sweet potato.

SWEET POTATO, VINE TOMATO, HALLOUMI & KALE TRAY BAKE

SERVES 2

2 small–medium sweet potatoes, halved and cut into wedges
1 tablespoon extra virgin olive oil
1 teaspoon ground sumac
60g (2oz/heaped ½ cup) pitted kalamata olives
50g (1¾oz) kale leaves, trimmed as necessary
2–3 stems vine-ripened cherry tomatoes
200g (7oz) halloumi cheese, cut into slices

Preheat the oven to 200°C/400°F/Gas 6.

Place the sweet potato wedges into a mixing bowl, drizzle with the extra virgin olive oil and then sprinkle with the sumac. Toss to combine, then place in a large roasting tray and scatter over the olives.

Roast in the preheated oven for 20 minutes or until the sweet potato wedges are just beginning to soften, then add the kale, cherry tomatoes and halloumi slices. Roast for a further 20 minutes or until the kale is charred, the tomatoes are blistered and the halloumi is a little golden. Remove from the oven and divide between 2 plates. Eat while still warm and the halloumi is soft.

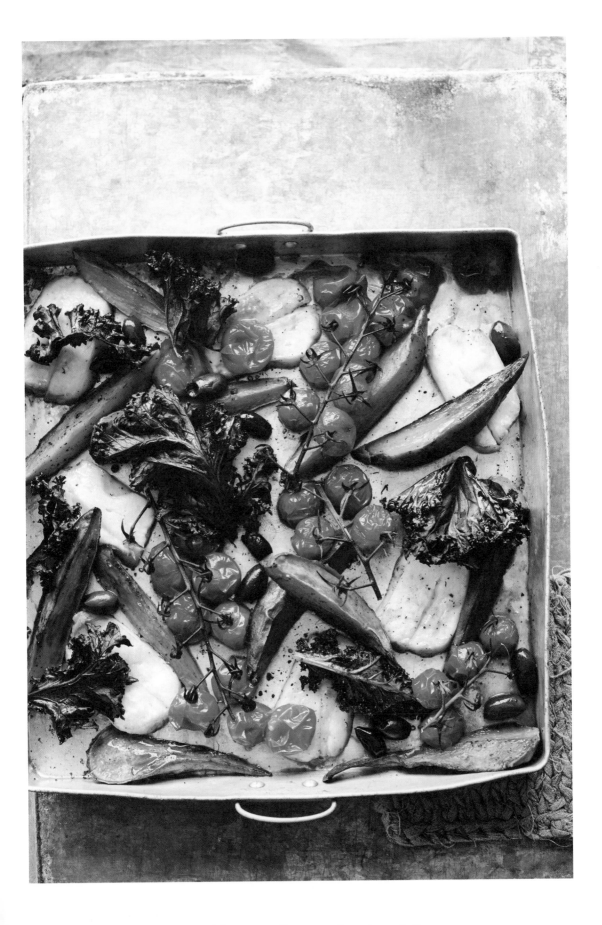

Making a good risotto brings me so much joy. I love the attention it demands and how intimate the cooking process becomes. Finding that perfect al dente grain and creamy texture is something I really enjoy.

SQUASH, SAGE & SPELT RISOTTO
with amaretti

SERVES 2–4

½ teaspoon ground cinnamon
a good pinch of dried chilli
    (hot pepper) flakes
½ teaspoon sea salt
¼ teaspoon cracked black pepper
6 tablespoons extra virgin olive oil
½ butternut squash, peeled,
    deseeded and cut into 2cm
    (¾in) dice
1 litre (35fl oz/4 cups)
    vegetable stock
1 celery stick, finely diced
150g (5½oz/scant 1 cup)
    pearled spelt, rinsed well
1 tablespoon mascarpone,
    or oat cream
1 tablespoon butter or coconut oil
20g (⅔oz/¼ cup) grated
    Parmesan cheese
a handful of rocket (arugula)
    leaves
4 large sage leaves
2–3 sweet almond (amaretti)
    biscuits, to serve (optional but
    recommended)

Preheat the oven to 200°C/400°F/Gas 6. Line a baking sheet with baking paper and set aside.

Stir the cinnamon, chilli flakes, salt and pepper together with 2 tablespoons of the olive oil to create a paste. Add the squash and toss to coat in the paste, then spread evenly over the baking sheet. Place the squash in the oven and roast for about 30 minutes, or until the pieces are soft and caramelized. Remove from the oven and put to one side.

While the squash is cooking, pour the stock into a saucepan and bring it to the boil. Then turn the heat down to a simmer.

Meanwhile, heat 2 more tablespoons of olive oil in a wide saucepan. Add the celery and sauté for a few minutes to soften, then add the spelt, stirring to coat. Add 1–2 ladles of the hot stock and lower the heat so the liquid is at a light simmer. Keep adding a little more stock as it is absorbed by the spelt. Taste after cooking for about 30 minutes. It should be softening, yet firm, and the risotto should be quite loose.

Lightly mash the squash pieces with a fork, then stir into the risotto. Continue to cook for a further 10 minutes, adding stock as needed, checking the spelt regularly – you want it to be cooked but still with a little bite. (You may not need all the stock.) Remove from the heat and stir through the mascarpone or oat cream, butter or coconut oil, and the Parmesan. The risotto should be loose and creamy. Stir through the rocket, cover the pan and leave the risotto to rest for a minute.

Meanwhile, heat a frying pan with the remaining olive oil. Gently fry the sage leaves for 1–2 minutes until crispy, then remove with a slotted spoon on to some kitchen paper.

Divide the risotto between 2 plates and just before serving, crush the amaretti over the top. Garnish with fried sage leaves.

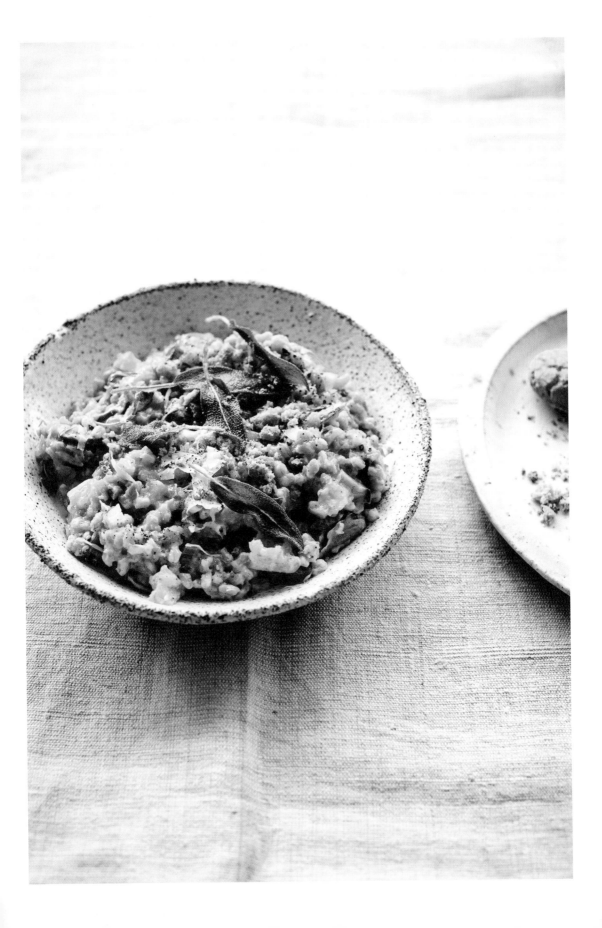

If you don't get through the whole squash in one sitting, you can freeze the slices and enjoy again as part of next weeks sacral chakra meals.

The miso savoy cabbage takes minutes to prepare, so you can turn it into a quick and easy meal for dinner.

STUFFED WHOLE SQUASH
with miso mustard savoy cabbage (v)

SERVES 4

1 butternut squash (about 1.5kg/3lb 5oz)
2 tablespoons extra virgin olive oil
1 celery stick, finely diced
20g (⅔oz/1 cup) parsley, finely chopped, plus extra to serve
1 teaspoon dried thyme
1 teaspoon rosemary, finely chopped
70g (2½oz/⅔ cup) sundried tomatoes in oil, drained
75g (2½oz/heaped ½ cup) cooked chestnuts
75g (2½oz/½ cup) dried apricots or dates, roughly chopped
50g (1¾oz/¼ cup) brown rice
2 pinches of ground allspice
350ml (12fl oz/1½ cups) vegetable stock
1½ teaspoons sea salt
cracked black pepper, to taste

FOR THE MISO MUSTARD SAVOY CABBAGE

1 tablespoon white miso paste
1 teaspoon tamari sauce
1 teaspoon Dijon mustard
1 tablespoon toasted sesame oil
½ teaspoon black sesame seeds
1 tablespoon maple syrup
2 teaspoons grated ginger
3 tablespoons extra virgin olive oil
½ savoy cabbage, thinly sliced

Wash the squash and cut it in half lengthways, then use a spoon to remove the seeds. Scrape out the flesh, making a gully for the stuffing along the full length. Collect the scooped-out flesh and finely chop. Add the 2 tablespoons of olive oil to a frying pan over medium heat. Add the celery, parsley, dried thyme and rosemary. Cook the squash flesh in the herbs for 10 minutes.

Chop the sundried tomatoes together with the chestnuts and dried apricots. Add to the pan along with the rice and allspice, and stir. Add the vegetable stock, sea salt and black pepper, and mix well. Cover and allow the rice to cook for 15–20 minutes, stirring occasionally. Check that all the liquid has been absorbed, then remove from the heat. It's okay if the rice is still a little al dente, as it will continue to cook once in the oven.

Preheat the oven to 200°C/400°F/Gas 6. Pack the stuffing tightly into the gully in the 2 squash halves, then press the halves back together and secure with kitchen twine. Rub the squash with oil, salt and pepper. Place on a large roasting tray lined with non-stick baking paper. Cover with foil and cook for 1 hour 45 minutes–2 hours, or until the squash is tender. Remove the foil, brush the squash with maple syrup and cook, brushing occasionally, for a further 15 minutes or until the squash is dark golden brown. Remove from the oven and let sit for 30 minutes.

While waiting, make the miso mustard savoy cabbage. Add the miso paste, tamari, Dijon mustard, sesame oil and seeds, maple syrup, ginger and 1 tablespoon water to a bowl and whisk, then set aside. Heat the olive oil in a large frying pan or wok. Add the cabbage and sauté for 6–8 minutes or until soft. Add the miso mustard sauce and stir to combine. Remove from the heat.

Divide the cabbage between serving plates, then cut the squash into thick slices and place on top. Sprinkle with chopped parsley.

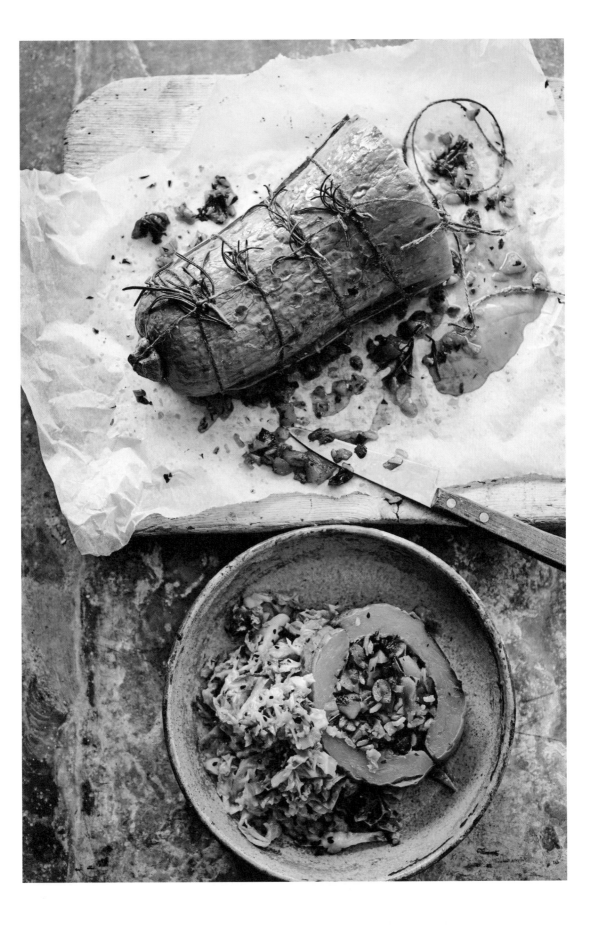

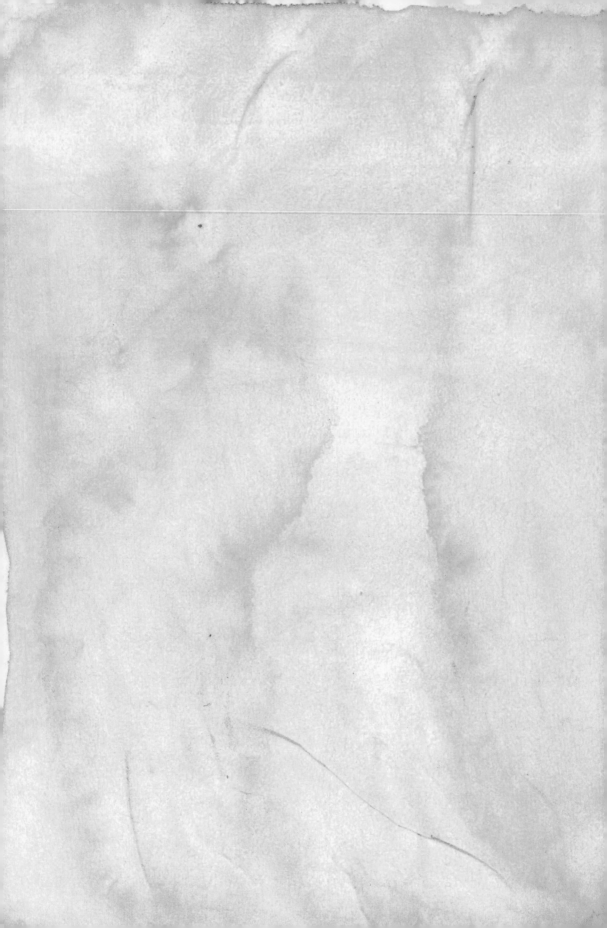

SOLAR PLEXUS CHAKRA
radiance

Key foods for the solar-plexus chakra:
YELLOW FOOD: pineapple, banana, passion fruit
COMPLEX CARBOHYDRATES: oats, beans and
pulses of all kinds, legumes such as
chickpeas, chestnut, corn
FRUITS & SWEETENERS: honey, dates, maple syrup
HERBS: lucuma, licorice, turmeric
B-VITAMIN-RICH FOOD TO BOOST METABOLISM:
nutritional yeast
Enjoy food that offers the most 'fuel/energy'
and avoid stimulating foods, such as caffeine
and refined sugars

Middle Eastern labneh is the rich, creamy, tangy sister to yoghurt that has been strained to the point where it becomes extra thick and spreadable. The yoghurt maintains all its probiotic properties while losing its excess liquid.

You can use labneh in sweet or savoury dishes and it makes a lovely probiotic substitute for cream cheese. The best yoghurt to make labneh is an organic, natural, full-fat variety, such as Greek yoghurt. The key is to make sure it hasn't had any refined-sugars added to ensure its probiotic quality.

Orange blossom adds a gorgeous, floral component to this dish, but if you don't have any in your pantry you can omit it and perhaps add some grated orange or lemon zest instead.

ORANGE BLOSSOM LABNEH
served with fruit-bread toast

SERVES 2

400g (14oz/1¾ cups) full-fat, natural yoghurt
2 teaspoons maple syrup, plus extra to serve (optional)
2 teaspoons orange blossom water
4 thick slices of fruit bread
1½ tablespoons pistachios, toasted and roughly chopped

Place a muslin (cheesecloth) inside a sieve sitting over a mixing bowl. If you don't have a cheesecloth, you can use 3 sheets of kitchen paper or a clean tea towel. Pour the yoghurt into the lined sieve, place in the fridge and allow to drip for a minimum of 3 hours or ideally overnight. It will thicken as it sits and the liquid drips away through the sieve.

Once strained, discard the liquid in the bowl and tip the thick yoghurt, now labneh, into a clean mixing bowl. Stir in the maple syrup and the orange blossom water.

Toast the slices of fruit bread, then spoon 2 tablespoons of labneh onto each piece of toast while still warm. Drizzle over a little more maple syrup, if desired. Scatter with pistachios and serve.

Store any leftover labneh in the fridge, covered, for up to 1 week.

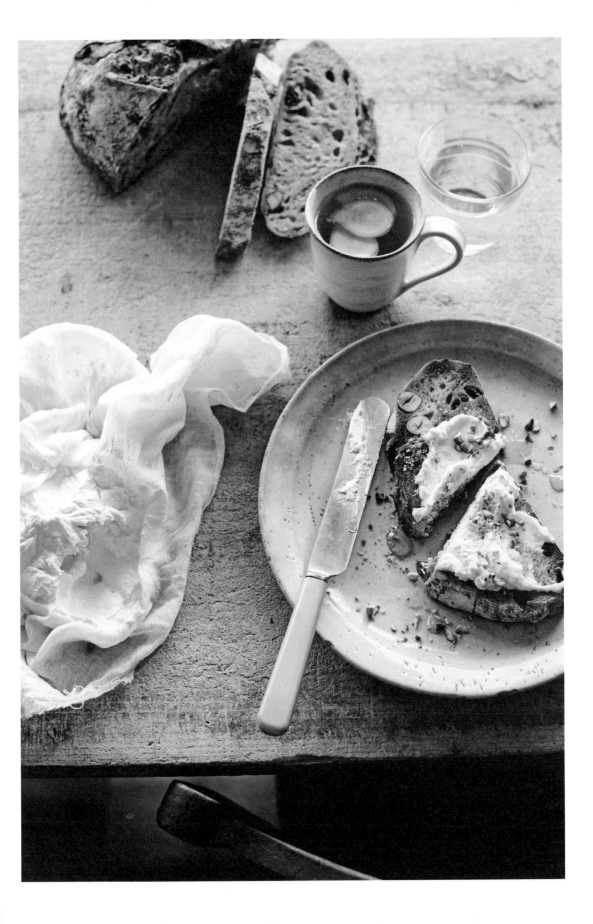

I often start my day off with fruit. Just plain and simple, straight-up berries, apricots, banana, mango, grapefruit or plums – whatever is seasonal and ripe at the time. It's the perfect way to start off the day with a dose of fibre and nutrients.

When I need a little more sustenance (on days I need fuel to get me all the way through to lunchtime), adding oats makes a good accompaniment to my daily fruit. I also love to add spices to my porridge and this gorgeously vibrant bowl with added turmeric powder just makes me feel so happy. In testing, I also tried this porridge with ground ginger which is also a lovely addition if you fancy a slightly spicier porridge.

SWEET MANGO & TURMERIC PORRIDGE BOWL (v)

SERVES 2

150g (5½oz/1½ cups)
   rolled oats
1 teaspoon ground turmeric
1 teaspoon ground cinnamon
480ml (16¾fl oz/2 cups) oat milk
   or milk of your choice
3 tablespoons maple syrup
1 tablespoon freshly squeezed
   lemon juice
½ mango, peeled, stoned and cut
   into long wedges
pulp from 1 passion fruit
5–6 macadamia nuts or nuts of
   your choice, roughly chopped

Add the oats, turmeric and cinnamon to a small saucepan, stir to combine, then add the milk and maple syrup. Place over a medium heat and slowly bring to a steady simmer, then simmer for 3–4 minutes, stirring occasionally. Once the oats are tender and cooked, remove from the heat and add the lemon juice. Stir to combine, then divide between 2 breakfast bowls.

To serve, top the porridge with the mango wedges and passion-fruit pulp, plus a sprinkle of chopped nuts.

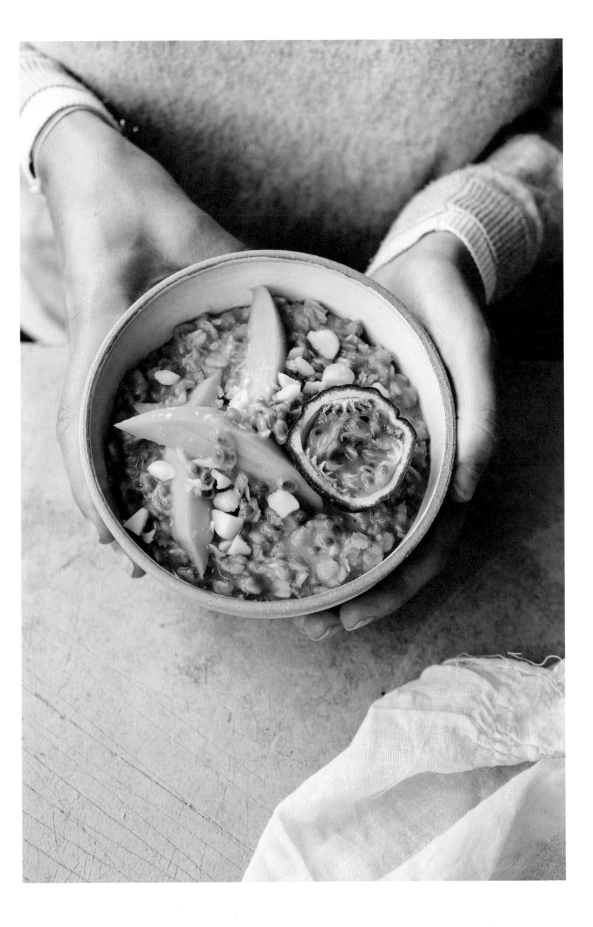

Make sure your ingredients are the freshest you can find and the tomatoes are ripe. I never store tomatoes in the fridge as their flavours deepen better at room temperature. This salad should be crisp, refreshing, salty and tart all at the same time. Dress it at the every last second before serving, otherwise it will start to wilt and swim in its own juices.

A REALLY GOOD FATTOUSH
with creamy butter-bean hummus (v)

SERVES 2

FOR THE HUMMUS

3½ tablespoons olive oil
3 thyme sprigs
1 x 400g (14oz) can butter beans (lima beans), rinsed
1 teaspoon ground cumin
2 tablespoons fresh lemon juice
½ teaspoon sea salt

FOR THE FATTOUSH

1 naan bread or wholemeal pita bread
1 tablespoon extra virgin olive oil
1 celery stick, thinly sliced
4 radishes, thinly sliced
12 vine tomatoes, halved
½ fennel bulb, trimmed
1 Lebanese cucumber
1 little gem (Bibb) lettuce, chopped
3 mint sprigs, leaves picked
4 parsley sprigs, leaves picked
seeds from ¼ pomegranate
¼ teaspoon ground sumac
cracked black pepper

FOR THE DRESSING

1 teaspoon ground sumac, soaked in 2 teaspoons warm water for 15 minutes
1½ tablespoons fresh lemon juice
1 tablespoon pomegranate molasses
1 teaspoon white wine vinegar
2 teaspoons finely chopped mint
4 tablespoons extra virgin olive oil
½ teaspoon sea salt

Begin by preparing the hummus. Heat the oil in a small saucepan on a medium heat, then very gently fry the thyme sprigs for 2–3 minutes until the oil becomes aromatic. Remove from the heat and discard the thyme sprigs. Tip the oil from the pan into a food processor with the beans, cumin, lemon juice and salt. Blitz until the mixture has the consistency of hummus, adding a little water to reach your preferred consistency.

Start the fattoush. Preheat the oven to 180°C/350°F/Gas 4, then bake the naan or pita bread for 5–7 minutes or until golden and toasted. Remove from the oven and allow to cool while you make the dressing.

To make the dressing combine the sumac with its soaking liquid, lemon juice, pomegranate molasses, white wine vinegar and mint in a small bowl. Gradually add the oil, whisking constantly until well blended. Season with the salt.

To complete the fattoush, chop the baked bread into bite-size pieces, place in a small mixing bowl, then drizzle with the olive oil. Toss to coat and season to taste with a little salt and pepper. Set aside.

Put the celery, radishes and halved tomatoes in a separate, larger mixing bowl. Using a peeler, peel thin slices of fennel into the bowl. Peel the cucumber, then slice it into half moons. Add to the mixing bowl along with the lettuce, mint, parsley and pomegranate seeds. Toss to combine and add three-quarters of the dressing, adding more dressing and salt, as needed. Add the naan bread pieces and toss once.

Divide the salad into bowls, sprinkle the sumac over and serve with a dollop of creamy butter-bean hummus.

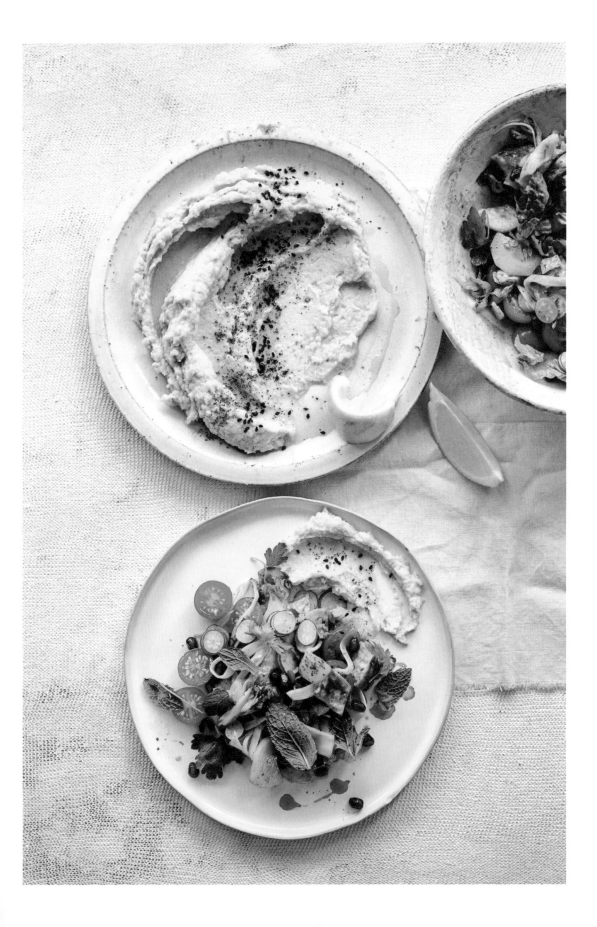

Sweet corn and black beans are two ingredients that pack a powerful energy punch. This salad really works well with some creamy avocado on the side for another texture dimension.

GRILLED LETTUCE, CORN & BLACK BEAN CHOP SALAD

SERVES 2

FOR THE SALAD

2 corn cobs (ears of corn), husks removed
200g (7oz/1⅓ cups) canned black beans, drained and rinsed
1 celery stick, trimmed and thinly sliced
1 baby cos or gem (Bibb) lettuce, quartered lengthways
½ tablespoon extra virgin olive oil
100g (3½oz) cherry tomatoes, halved
1 ripe avocado, pitted, peeled and sliced

FOR THE CORIANDER YOGHURT DRESSING

140g (5oz/generous ½ cup) full-fat, natural Greek yoghurt, or yoghurt of your choice
2 tablespoons freshly squeezed lime juice
3 coriander sprigs (cilantro), leaves picked and finely chopped
sea salt and cracked black pepper

TO SERVE

1 tablespoon pine nuts/kernels or cashews, toasted
2 lime wedges

Preheat a ridged griddle (char-grill) pan over high heat and cook the corn cobs for 10–12 minutes, turning regularly. (You can also do this on a barbecue.) Slice the charred kernels off the cob by placing a fork in one end of the cob and standing it up on the other end. Use a sharp knife to carefully slice down the side of the cob between the husk and corn kernels. Place the corn kernels, black beans and celery in a mixing bowl and toss to combine.

Brush the lettuce with the olive oil and cook on the same griddle pan for 2 minutes each side or until charred.

To make the coriander yoghurt dressing, put the yoghurt, lime juice and coriander in a bowl and stir to combine. Season with salt and pepper.

Divide the charred lettuce between 2 serving plates, top with the corn and bean mixture, then add the tomatoes and avocado, and the coriander and yoghurt dressing. To serve, sprinkle with the toasted pine nuts or cashews and add a wedge of lime alongside. Enjoy immediately.

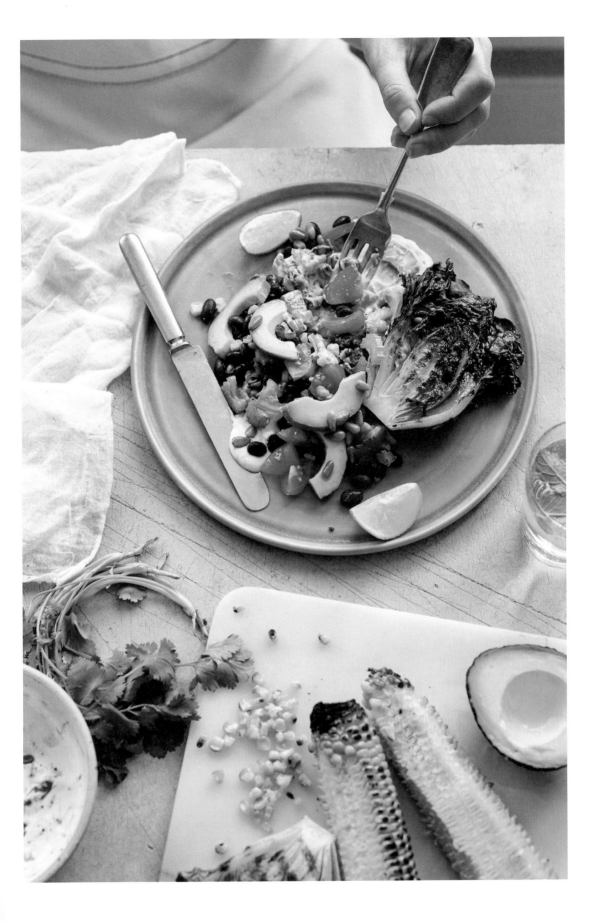

These wraps are easy to make and are quite like crêpes. Use a non-stick pan and pay attention while cooking, as they are thin and won't need long. As with most chillis, this is best made the day before eating. The recipe is also good for freezing in portions (even the wraps, between sheets of baking paper).

TURMERIC BURRITO
with mexican bean chilli & cauli rice (v)

SERVES 8

½ head of cauliflower, chopped into florets
1 avocado, pitted, peeled and cut into thin slices
sour cream or yoghurt (vegan if necessary)
2 lime wedges

FOR THE BEAN CHILLI

2 celery sticks, finely diced
2 tablespoons extra virgin olive oil
2 tablespoons tomato purée (paste)
2 teaspoons ground cumin
1 teaspoon smoked paprika
½ teaspoon dried chilli (hot pepper) flakes
½ teaspoon ground coriander
½ teaspoon ground turmeric
1 x 400g (14oz) can black beans, drained and rinsed
1 x 400g (14oz) can red kidney beans, drained and rinsed
1 x 400g (14oz) can black eyed beans, drained and rinsed
1 x 400g (14oz) can chopped tomatoes
1 vegetable stock cube
sea salt and cracked black pepper

FOR THE TURMERIC WRAPS

2 tablespoons ground flaxseed
175g (6oz/heaped 1¼ cups) chickpea (gram) flour
1 teaspoon ground turmeric
2 teaspoons ground cumin
½ teaspoon of salt
2 tablespoons olive oil

For the chilli, put the olive oil and celery in a large saucepan. Sauté over a medium heat until translucent, about 2–3 minutes. Add the tomato purée and spices and stir to completely combine. Add the all beans, the tomatoes, stock cube and 250ml (9fl oz/1 cup) water. Stir again and lower the heat to medium–low. Cover and gently simmer for 20 minutes. Check for seasoning, then cook without the lid for an extra 20 minutes. Allow to rest.

To make the wraps, whisk together the ground flaxseed and 4 tablespoons warm water in a bowl. Let sit for 5 minutes to thicken slightly. Add the chickpea flour, spices, 250ml (9fl oz/ 1 cup) water, salt and olive oil. Whisk until there are no lumps. The mixture should be about the consistency of a thin pancake batter. Heat a lightly greased 23cm (9in) frying pan over medium heat. Pour about 3 tablespoons of batter into the pan and swirl to coat the base. Cook the wrap for 1–2 minutes or until you see the edges start to dry out. You will easily be able to slide your spatula underneath the wrap when the bottom is fully cooked and ready to be flipped. Flip and cook for an additional 30–60 seconds, then remove from the pan and repeat for all the other wraps. You should get 8 out of the mixture.

To make the cauli rice, place the cauliflower in a lidded pan with 100ml (3½fl oz/scant ½ cup) water or into a steamer and steam over a pan of boiling water for 4–5 minutes, until just tender but not soft. Transfer the cauliflower to a food processor and pulse until it resembles small grains of rice. Put in a serving bowl.

To assemble your burrito, place a turmeric wrap on a plate, place 1–2 tablespoons of the cauli rice in the centre, and add 2–3 tablespoons of the bean chilli. Add a few avocado slices, a dollop of yoghurt and a squeeze of lime. Fold the tortilla up into a burrito and enjoy while still warm.

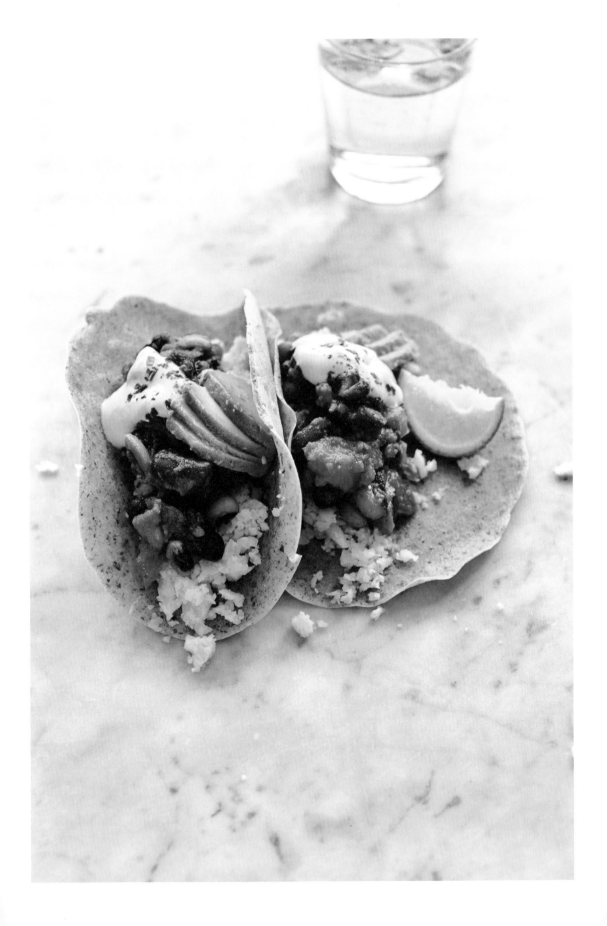

Perfect for a little lunchtime pick-me-up, this salad is fresh, vibrant and packs a mild kick at the end from the warmth of the kimchi spices. If you can't find store-bought kimchi with turmeric and carrot flavouring, you can buy a regular kimchi variety and add some grated fresh turmeric and carrot to it.

PEARL BARLEY, TURMERIC & CARROT KIMCHI SALAD
with sweet paprika cashews (v)

SERVES 2

110g (3¾oz/heaped ½ cup) pearl barley, quinoa or freekeh
130g (4¾oz/scant 1 cup) store-bought turmeric & carrot kimchi, or other store-bought kimchi (make sure it is vegan)
1 tablespoon apple cider vinegar
1 tablespoon extra virgin olive oil
50g (1¾oz/½ cup) mangetout (snow peas), trimmed and blanched
50g (1¾oz/½ cup) sugar snap peas, trimmed and blanched
50g (1¾oz/heaped ⅓ cup) edamame beans
1 small courgette (zucchini), julienned
5 coriander (cilantro) sprigs, leaves picked and roughly torn
sea salt and cracked black pepper
25g (1oz) Smoked Paprika, Chilli & Lime Chia Seed Mixed Nuts (see page 182), to serve

Put the barley, quinoa or freekeh in a medium saucepan with 320ml (11fl oz/1⅓ cups) water, place over a high heat and bring to the boil. Reduce the heat to medium and simmer for 20–25 minutes (10–15 for quinoa) or until tender and the liquid is absorbed. Remove from the heat and set aside to cool.

Squeeze the kimchi to remove the excess liquid, reserving the liquid in a small bowl.

To make a dressing, place the vinegar, olive oil and 2 tablespoons of the reserved kimchi liquid in a small bowl, season to taste with salt and pepper and stir to combine.

Place the kimchi, mangetout, sugar snap peas, edamame, courgette and cooked grain into a large mixing bowl. Add the coriander and dressing and gently toss together.

Divide the salad between 2 serving plates and top with the mixed nuts to serve.

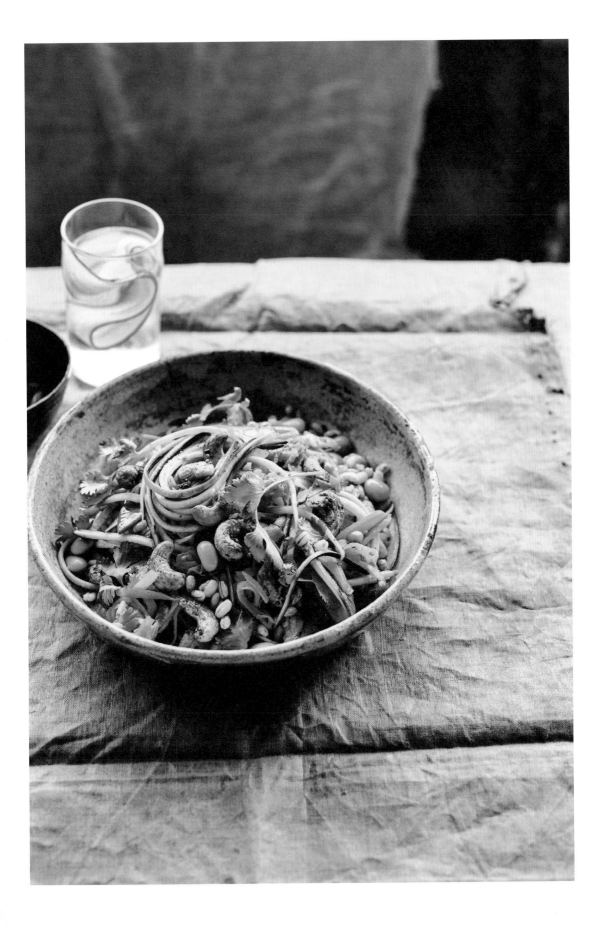

You may think of polenta as quite a bland ingredient, but when you add robust flavours, such as green olives, polenta takes on a whole new life. You can also add finely chopped sundried tomatoes and basil leaves to the base instead of the olives for another flavour sensation.

SICILIAN GREEN OLIVE POLENTA PIZZAS

with squash, goat's cheese, green pesto & padrón peppers

SERVES 4

FOR THE POLENTA PIZZAS

625ml (21½fl oz/2½ cups) vegetable stock
120g (4¼oz/¾ cup) polenta (cornmeal)
2 tablespoons extra virgin olive oil, plus extra for drizzling over the squash
1 tablespoon apple cider vinegar
4 tablespoons finely chopped parsley
110g (3¾oz/heaped 1 cup) pitted Sicilian green olives, roughly chopped
sea salt and cracked black pepper

TOPPINGS

600g (1lb 5oz) butternut squash, peeled and cut into slim wedges
120g (4¼oz) padrón peppers
120g (4¼oz/1 cup) roughly crumbled goat's cheese
40g (1½oz/scant 1 cup) rocket (arugula) leaves
4 tablespoons Green Vegan Pesto (see Courgette Ribbon, White Bean Smash & Pesto Bruschetta on page 108)
2 teaspoons sunflower seeds

Preheat the oven to 200°C/400°F/Gas 6. Line 2 round pizza baking sheets with baking paper. Begin by roasting the squash. Distribute the squash pieces evenly over a large baking sheet, drizzle with olive oil and sprinkle with sea salt. Roast in the oven for 25–30 minutes or until golden and crisp. Remove from the oven and set aside. Leave the oven on.

To make the pizza bases, in a wide saucepan, bring the vegetable stock to the boil. Reduce the heat to a simmer and add the polenta and olive oil, whisking continuously to avoid lumps of polenta forming. Cook, stirring regularly, until the polenta is soft and smooth, about 10 minutes. Turn off the heat, add the vinegar and season to taste. Fold the parsley and olives through the polenta. Check the seasoning and add extra salt if needed. Polenta is quite bland by nature, so don't be shy.

Place half the polenta mixture into the centre of each prepared pizza baking sheet. Use a silicone spatula to smooth it into rounds about 1.5cm (⅝in) thick. Bake the pizza bases for 30 minutes or until crispy on the edges. Remove from the oven and check that the centre of each pizza base is a little crispy too. If not, keep baking until the centre is cooked and crispy.

Place half the roasted squash, padrón peppers and goat's cheese onto each pizza. Return to the oven and bake for a further 10–15 minutes or until the cheese has melted and begun to turn golden.

Remove the pizzas from the oven and add some rocket leaves, a drizzle of green pesto and a sprinkle of sunflower seeds. Serve hot.

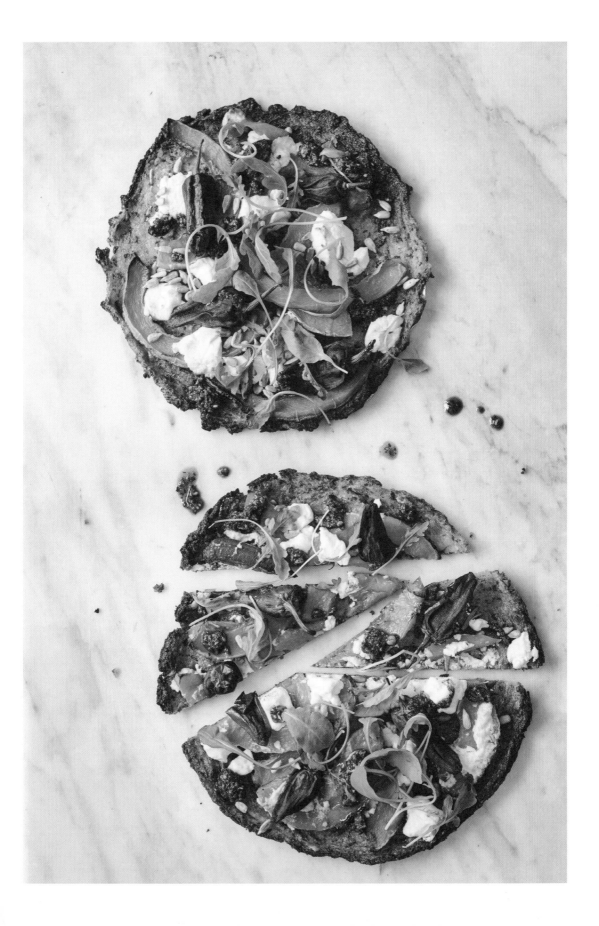

If there is one easy weekday meal I love to make over and over again, it's this one. The combination of turmeric with cauliflower isn't new, but it just works so well. The ginger adds casual warmth without dominating, while the lemon and herbs is refreshing and cooling. This is a stew for any season.

GOLDEN CAULIFLOWER CHICKPEA STEW
with spelt, parsnip & rosemary flatbread (v)

SERVES 2

FOR THE FLATBREAD

75g (2½oz/heaped ½ cup) spelt flour, plus extra for kneading
40g (1½oz/⅓ cup) chickpea (gram) flour
2 tablespoons extra virgin olive oil
1 teaspoon baking powder
1 teaspoon sea salt flakes
200g (7oz, roughly 2 small) parsnips, peeled and thinly sliced using a mandoline
25g (1oz/¼ cup) Parmesan shavings (optional, if vegan)
4–5 rosemary sprigs, leaves picked
sea salt and cracked black pepper

FOR THE GOLDEN STEW

2 tablespoons olive oil
1 celery stick, washed and diced
2 tablespoons fresh grated ginger
1 teaspoon ground turmeric
1 vegetable stock cube
½ head cauliflower, chopped into florets
400ml (14fl oz/1¾ cups) can full-fat coconut milk
1 x 400g (14oz) can chickpeas (garbanzo beans), rinsed and drained
½ courgette (zucchini), sliced
20g (⅔oz/1 cup) each of parsley and coriander (cilantro), roughly chopped
zest and juice of 1 lemon

Begin by making the flatbread. Preheat the oven to 220°C/425°F/Gas 7. Line a baking sheet with baking paper. Set aside.

Place the spelt and chickpea flours in a large bowl. Add 1 tablespoon of the olive oil, and the baking powder, salt and 80ml (2½fl oz/5½ tablespoons) water. Mix well to combine. Alternatively, add all the ingredients to your food processor and, using the bread paddle, process until a dough forms.

Turn the dough out onto a flour-dusted surface and knead until the dough is smooth. Using a floured rolling pin, roll the dough out to a 40 x 20cm (16 x 8in) rectangle and place on the prepared baking sheet. The flatbread should be roughly ¾cm (⅓in) thick. Top with the parsnip slices, Parmesan, if using, and rosemary, drizzle with the remaining 1 tablespoon olive oil and sprinkle with salt and black pepper. Bake for 25 minutes or until golden brown and crisp.

To make the golden stew, put the olive oil in a large heavy-based saucepan and place over a low heat. Add the celery, 1 tablespoon of the grated ginger and the turmeric, and sauté for 2–3 minutes. Now add 240ml (8fl oz/1 cup) water, the stock cube and cauliflower florets, increase the heat to medium and bring to a steady simmer. Simmer for 10 minutes, then add the coconut milk, chickpeas and courgette. Simmer for a further 5 minutes. Remove from the heat, and stir through the remaining 1 tablespoon ginger, along with the parsley, coriander and lemon zest and juice. Check the seasoning and serve piping hot with a slice of the flatbread.

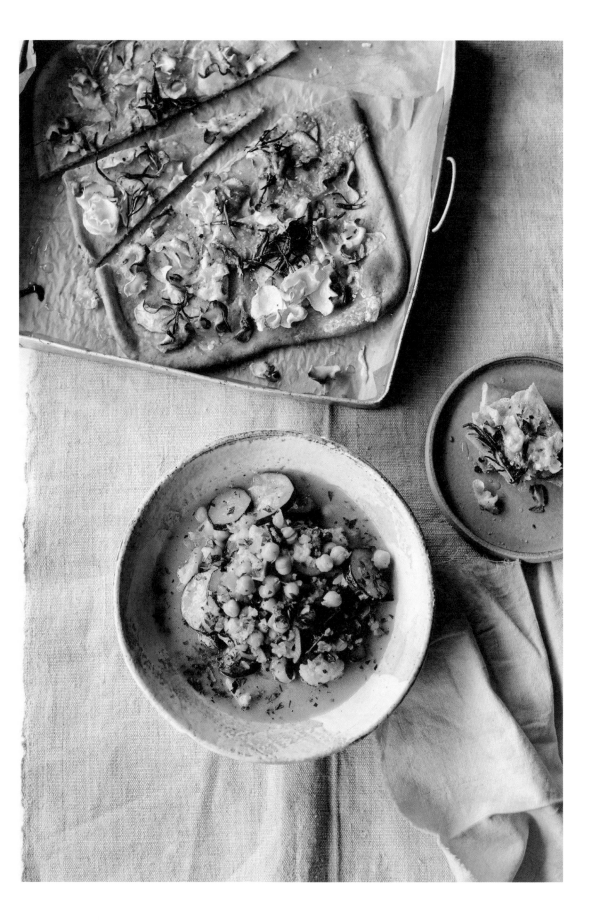

I love food that means you can put down your cutlery and use your hands. Tacos are so tactile and often best created in the palm of your hand and eaten as you hover over a plate.

The use of polenta in these corn fritters is a genius way to help bring all the ingredients together without making everything dry from the addition of wheat flour.

SOFT SHELL TACOS WITH CORN FRITTERS
& zesty green goddess dressing (v)

SERVES 2

2 large tomatoes, diced
8 baby gem (Bibb) lettuce leaves

FOR THE CORN FRITTERS

1 vegetable stock cube
100g (3½oz/⅔ cup) quick-cook polenta (cornmeal)
260g (9¼oz/scant 2 cups) frozen corn kernels, thawed
1 celery stick, finely diced
a good pinch of dried chilli (hot pepper) flakes
1 tablespoon chopped dill
1 tablespoon chopped coriander (cilantro)
60ml (2fl oz/¼ cup) extra virgin olive oil
black sesame seeds (optional)

FOR THE WRAPS

2 tablespoons ground flaxseed
175g (6oz/heaped 1¼ cups) chickpea (gram) flour
1 teaspoon ground turmeric
2 teaspoons ground cumin
½ teaspoon of salt
2 tablespoons extra virgin olive oil

FOR THE DRESSING

flesh of 1 avocado
2 tablespoons coriander (cilantro) leaves, plus extra
zest and juice of 1 lime
a pinch of sea salt
2 tablespoons extra virgin olive oil
sea salt and cracked black pepper

Preheat the oven to 180°C/350°F/Gas 4. Line a baking sheet with baking paper and set aside. For the corn fritters, put the stock cube and 300ml (10½fl oz/1¼ cups) water into a saucepan and place over a medium heat. Bring to a light simmer and dissolve the stock cube into the water. Add the polenta and stir continuously for 2 minutes or until the polenta thickens and absorbs the liquid. Remove from the heat, add all the remaining fritter ingredients except the sesame seeds, and stir. Spoon the fritter mixture out and create patties on the baking sheet. Sprinkle a few sesame seeds over each fritter. Bake for 15 minutes or until slightly golden. Remove from the oven and keep warm.

For the wraps, whisk together the flaxseeds and 4 tablespoons warm water in a bowl and let sit for 5 minutes to thicken slightly. Add the chickpea flour, spices, salt, olive oil and 250ml (9fl oz/ 1 cup) water, and whisk until there are no lumps. The mixture should be roughly the consistency of a thin pancake batter. Preheat a lightly greased 15cm (6in) frying pan over medium heat. Pour about 2 tablespoons of batter into the pan and swirl to coat the base. Cook the wrap for 1–2 minutes or until the edges start to dry out. Flip and cook for an extra 30 seconds– 1 minute, then remove from pan and repeat for all other wraps. You should be able to make about 12 from the mixture.

For the dressing, place all ingredients in a high speed blender or food processor with 60ml (2fl oz/¼ cup) water and blend until smooth. Taste for seasoning and transfer to small serving bowl.

To serve, place a wrap on each serving plate, place a lettuce leaf and 2 corn fritters in the middle, then top with chopped tomatoes, a drizzle of dressing and some coriander leaves. Serve and enjoy. (The fritters can be frozen, as can the wraps if placed between sheets of baking paper.)

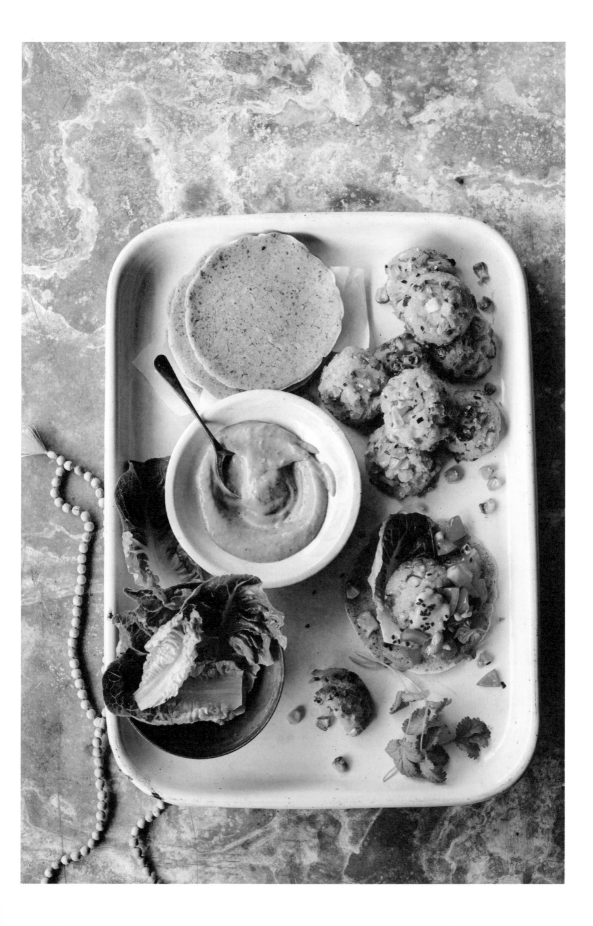

HEART CHAKRA
love

Key foods for the heart chakra:
GREEN FOOD: broccoli, green herbs,
asparagus, courgette, cucumber, lettuce,
edamame, peas, green beans
Eat highly nutritious, phytonutrient-dense food,
such as matcha, spirulina, moringa,
wheatgrass, barleygrass
LEAFY GREEN VEGETABLES:
kale, spinach, chard, rocket
HEALTHY FATS: avocado, nuts and seeds
Preparation methods, such as juices and smoothies
for quick absorption of nutrients
Enjoy food made with love and avoid stimulating
foods, such as caffeine and refined sugars

Aren't overnight oats just the most convenient breakfast idea ever?! Perfect for when breakfast needs to be on-the-go and, best of all, you finally get to use those recycled jars you keep accumulating on your kitchen sideboard.

The best oats used for overnight soaking recipes are the jumbo rolled oats, not the steel cut or 'quick' oat varieties. The oats soften a lot overnight, so in order for the dish to maintain some texture, it's best to use the best-quality jumbo oats you can find.

GREEN GLOW OVERNIGHT OATS
(v)

SERVES 2

150g (5½oz/1½ cups) jumbo
  rolled oats
50g (1¾oz/1 cup) coconut flakes
  or (⅔ cup) desiccated (dried
  shredded) coconut
50g (1¾oz/⅓ cup) currants
40g (1½oz/scant ¼ cup)
  pumpkin seeds
40g (1½oz/scant ¼ cup)
  sunflower seeds
2 teaspoons matcha powder
440ml (15½fl oz/scant 2 cups)
  vegan milk of your choice,
  plus extra to loosen
2 tablespoons maple syrup
blueberries, to serve

Combine all the dry ingredients a mixing bowl. Pour over the milk, cover and refrigerate overnight, or for at least 4 hours.

In the morning, add the maple syrup and some more milk to help loosen the mixture. Enjoy topped with some blueberries.

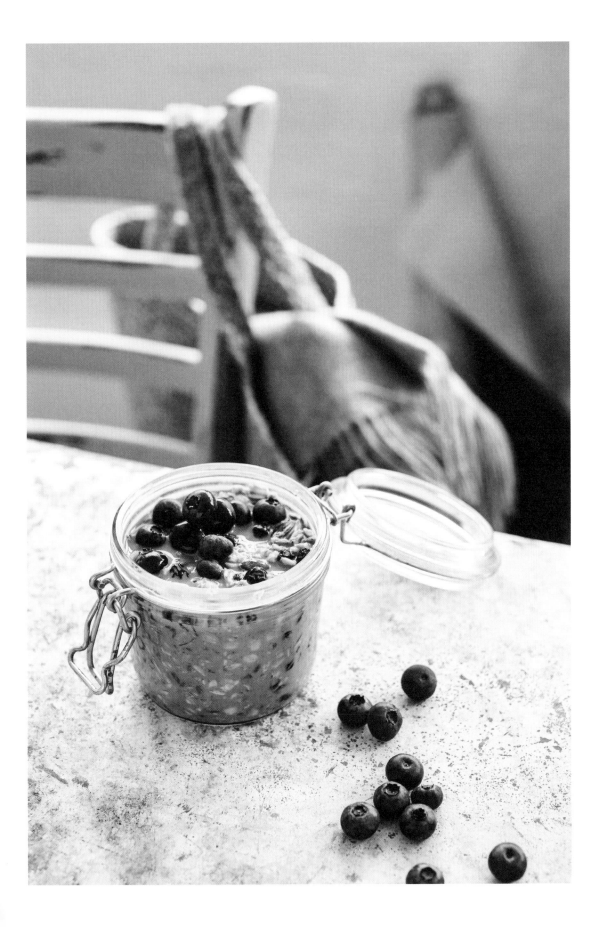

This green smoothie bowl will nourish your body and transport your mind to the lush green rainforests of Bali, conjuring up all the yoga retreat vibes that island is so well known for.

If you want to pack even more green vegetables into this smoothie bowl, you can substitute the mango for cucumber or courgette instead, but I think the mango adds such a lovely hint of summer and complements the coconut so well.

I find that spinach blends smoother than kale – especially if you are not using a Vitamix-like blender – but you could use kale instead if you like. Frozen spinach is also fine here. You could also add a protein powder of your choice, if you desire.

GREEN SMOOTHIE BOWL
(v)

SERVES 2

FOR THE SMOOTHIE BOWL
240ml (8fl oz/1 cup)
   coconut water
2 tablespoons coconut butter
2 handfuls baby spinach
1 teaspoon moringa, wheatgrass
   or barley grass powder
250g (9oz/heaped 2 cups) frozen
   mango pieces
freshly squeezed juice of ½ lime
diced flesh of 2 avocados, frozen
2 ripe bananas, peeled and cut
   into 2cm (¾in) slices and frozen

FOR THE TOPPINGS
(ALL OPTIONAL)
toasted coconut flakes
hulled hemp seeds
green apple slices
slices of kiwi fruit (golden
   if possible)
mango wedges
kumquat slices

Begin by adding the coconut water, coconut butter, spinach and moringa, wheatgrass or barley grass powder to a blender or food processor. Blend on high speed for 1 minute. Add the remaining smoothie ingredients and blend on high speed until smooth. You may need to use the blender paddle or a silicon spatula to make sure all the ingredients are blended.

Divide the smoothie bowl contents between 2 bowls and top with desired toppings. Enjoy immediately with a spoon.

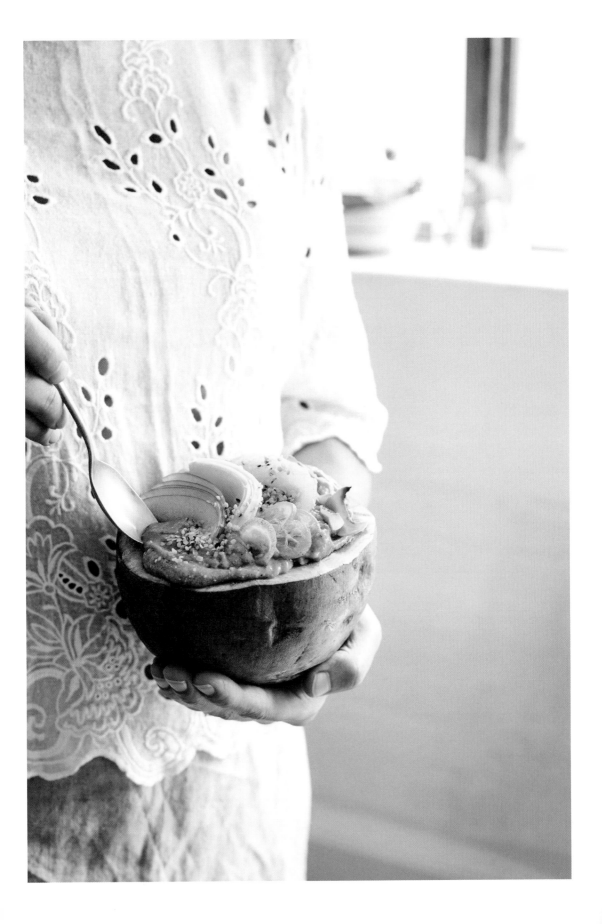

When avocado on toast gets repetitive, this is what happens in my kitchen – I start getting creative with what can enhance the humble avocado!

COCONUT CASHEW CREAM CHEESE CROSTINI
topped with edamame smash & pickled carrots (v)

SERVES 2

FOR THE PICKLED CARROTS

2 carrots, peeled and finely shredded
2 tablespoons rice wine vinegar

FOR THE COCONUT CASHEW CREAM CHEESE

100g (3½oz/heaped ¾ cup) cashews, soaked overnight, rinsed and drained
25g (1oz) fresh coconut flesh, or coconut flakes soaked for 15 minutes in warm water and drained
1 tablespoon sweet white miso paste
1 tablespoon nutritional yeast flakes
freshly squeezed juice of ½ lemon
1 teaspoon maple or agave syrup
a pinch of sea salt

FOR THE EDAMAME SMASH

1 avocado, peeled and pitted
4 basil sprigs, leaves picked
1 tablespoon chopped chives
freshly squeezed juice of ½ lemon
80ml (2½floz/⅓ cup) extra virgin olive oil
150g (5½oz/heaped 1 cup) frozen podded edamame beans, thawed
sea salt and cracked black pepper

TO SERVE

4 slices of rye bread, toasted
a pinch of dried chilli (hot pepper) flakes

Begin by pickling the carrots. Place the carrot and vinegar in a medium bowl and toss to combine. Set aside to pickle for 10 minutes, stirring occasionally.

To make the cream cheese, add all ingredients to the bowl of a food processor and process. Add up to 5 tablespoons water, a spoonful at a time, to reach a very smooth consistency.

To make the edamame smash, place the avocado, basil, chives, lemon juice and olive oil into a food processor. Process until smooth, then add the edamame and pulse to incorporate into the mixture until you reach a consistency you like. I like mine with small chunky pieces of edamame to add a little texture. Season to taste and set aside.

To serve, spread a layer of coconut cashew cream cheese over each rye toast, place a dollop of the edamame smash on top, then sprinkle with some pickled carrots and chilli flakes.

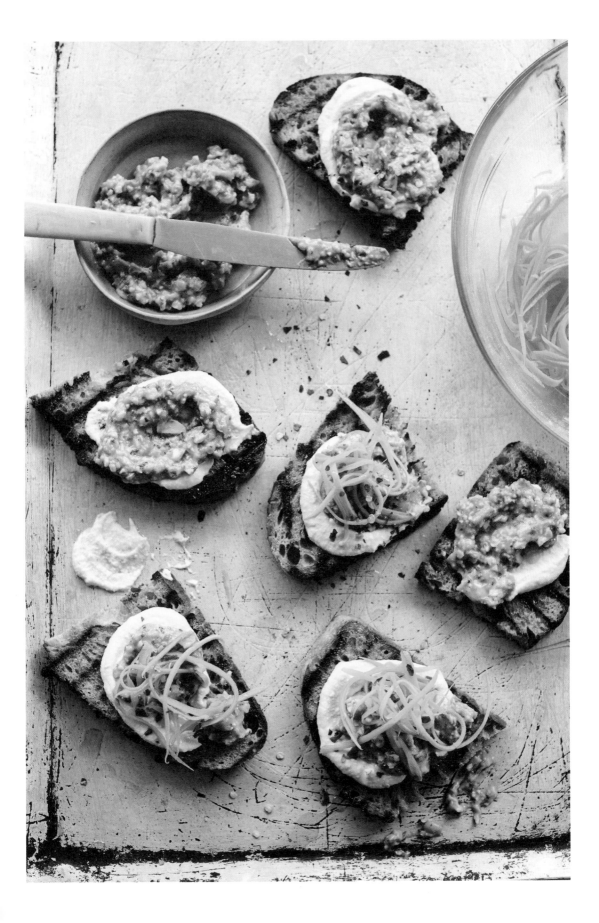

Crisp and light are the best way I can describe this salad – and delicate, too, due to the coconut yoghurt dressing, which seems to lift it to a mouth-puckering, smooth citrus sensation.

There is a lot to love about this salad (which is one that should be eaten immediately): the plump, sprouted mung beans that taste somewhat sweet and so satisfying to bite into; the crisp cucumber, lettuce and sugar snaps; and the freshness of the mint and coriander.

I never want my recipes to seem complex or unachievable and a salad like this is meant to remind us that fresh, simple ingredients put together well can be just as satisfying as a meal that we had to labour over. Sometimes simple is sophisticated, too.

SPROUTED MUNG BEAN SLAW
with fennel, cucumber, edamame & mint (v)

SERVES 2

FOR THE SALAD

50g (1¾oz/¼ cup) mung beans
½ cucumber, washed
1 fennel bulb
½ baby gem (Bibb) lettuce, leaves separated
70g (2½oz/½ cup) edamame beans
60g (2oz/heaped ½ cup) sugar snap peas, cut in half on a sharp angle
3–4 mint sprigs, leaves picked
3–4 coriander (cilantro) sprigs, leaves picked

FOR THE DRESSING

100g (3½oz/scant ½ cup) coconut yoghurt
zest of 1 lime
1 tablespoon freshly squeezed lime juice
sea salt and cracked black pepper

Two days in advance, soak your mung beans overnight (or for up to 8 hours) in enough water to cover them by at least 3cm (1¼in). Once soaked and you will be able to see that some of the bean skins have started to crack and the beans will have swollen. Drain and wash, then allow the beans to sit in the colander, covered with a kitchen towel, until little white shoots start to appear. It should take no more than a full day. If they haven't sprouted yet, rinse them again, cover and wait until they have sprouted. Sprouts take longer in the cooler months, so you may want to leave your colander in a warmer environment to speed up the process.

To make the salad, using a mandoline, thinly slice the cucumber into thin rounds. Then, thinly slice the fennel bulb using the same mandoline setting and place both ingredients in a mixing bowl. If you don't have a mandoline, use a sharp knife. Add the lettuce leaves, sprouted mung beans and half the edamame beans, sugar snap peas, and mint and coriander leaves.

In a small mixing bowl, mix all the dressing ingredients together. Pour the dressing over the salad and stir to coat.

Divide the salad between 2 serving plates, then sprinkle the remaining edamame, sugar snap peas, and mint and coriander leaves over the top. Serve straightaway.

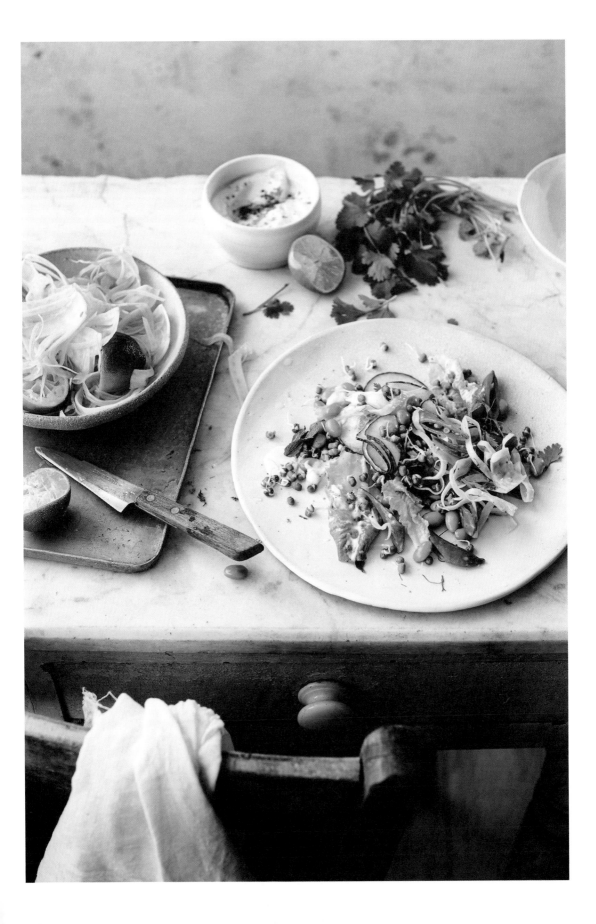

Elevating boring old toast into a truly nourishing, light meal, this easy-to-prepare, fresh flavour hit is protein-rich and bursting with green goodness. And that vegan pesto is just magic!

COURGETTE RIBBON, WHITE BEAN SMASH & PESTO BRUSCHETTA (v)

SERVES 2

1 large courgette (zucchini), thinly
   sliced into ribbons
1 x 400g (14oz) can cannellini
   beans, rinsed and drained
4 slices sourdough bread, toasted
sea salt flakes, to serve
2 lime wedges, to serve

FOR THE VEGAN PESTO

1 large bunch basil leaves,
   plus extra to serve
1 small bunch coriander
   (cilantro) leaves
30g (1oz/¼ cup) pine nuts/
   kernels, toasted
35g (1oz/¼ cup) raw
   pistachio nuts
120ml (4fl oz/½ cup) extra virgin
   olive oil, plus extra to drizzle
¾ teaspoon sea salt

To make the vegan pesto, place all the ingredients into a food processor and blitz until smooth. Set aside.

Place the courgette ribbons and beans in a large bowl, add a quarter of the pesto and toss to coat.

Divide the remaining pesto between the toasts, spreading it over the bread, then top with the courgette ribbons and beans. Drizzle with olive oil, scatter over some extra basil leaves and sea salt flakes and serve with lime wedges.

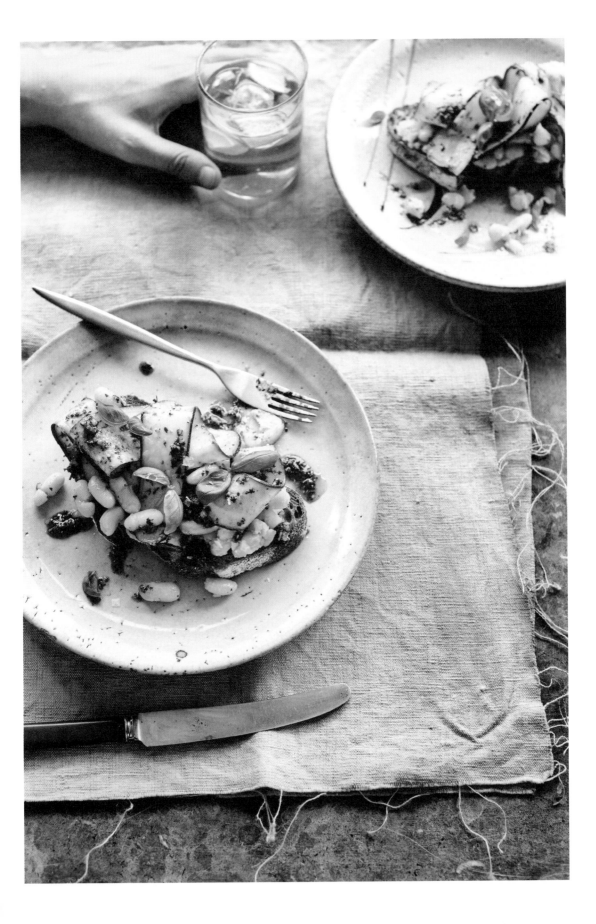

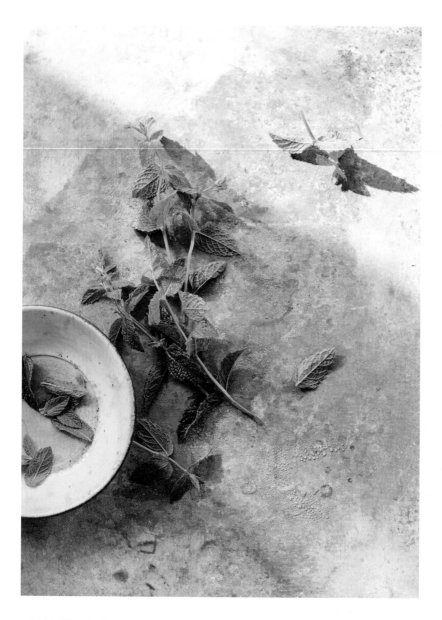

THE HEART CHAKRA IS CONNECTED TO HEALING AND LOVING ON ALL LEVELS (EMOTIONAL, MENTAL, PHYSICAL), WHILE HAVING THE ABILITY TO PROPERLY PROCESS YOUR EMOTIONS. IF YOU REGULARLY EXPERIENCE PROBLEMATIC OR DRAINING RELATIONSHIPS, OR FIND YOU HAVE A DIFFICULT TIME CONNECTING WITH PEOPLE IN A MEANINGFUL WAY, IT'S POSSIBLE THAT YOUR HEART CHAKRA IS OUT OF BALANCE.

OTHER SIGNS OF IMBALANCE INCLUDE SHYNESS, LACK OF EMPATHY, CO-DEPENDENCY, NEEDING VALIDATION FOR FULFILMENT, JEALOUSY, JUDGEMENT, LOW SELF-ESTEEM, BEING CRITICAL OR CONTROLLING, SUSPICIOUSNESS, FEELING POSSESSIVE, BEING AFRAID TO LET GO OF EMOTIONAL HURT, DEFENSIVENESS, AND DISTRUST.

You always need to have a healthy five-minute recipe up your sleeve and this is mine that I would like to share with you. This will take you only as long as it takes to put the ingredients into your blender and boil the kettle. Pour straight from the blender into a bowl and sit down to a meal in less time than it would have taken you to walk the aisle of a supermarket looking for a healthy ready-meal.

I think peas lend themselves to most herbs, so if you don't have any mint to hand, then try the basil you have growing next to your kitchen window. Coriander, thyme and tarragon will also work. The cannellini beans add a really lovely thickness to the soup, but you can use haricot or butter beans if you prefer.

FIVE-MINUTE PEA & MINT SOUP (v)

SERVES 2

400g (14oz/2⅔ cup)
    frozen peas
1 x 400g (14oz) can
    cannellini beans
1 vegetable stock cube
10g (⅓ oz/½ cup) mint leaves,
    leaves picked

Place all the ingredients into a blender with 500ml (17fl oz/ 2 cups) boiling water. Blend on high speed for 2–3 minutes.

Taste for seasoning, then add to a medium saucepan and warm through. Pour into 2 serving bowls and enjoy.

Is there anything more satisfying than a bowl of freshly made pasta served with a simple sauce and a smattering of cheese?

FLAXSEED LINGUINE
with asparagus pesto, burrata & basil oil

SERVES 2

FOR THE FLAXSEED
LINGUINE

2 tablespoons ground flaxseed
120ml (4fl oz/½ cup)
  filtered water
150g (5½oz/heaped 1 cup)
  pasta flour of your choice
a large pinch of sea salt
1 teaspoon extra virgin olive oil

FOR THE ASPARAGUS PESTO

100g (3½oz) asparagus, trimmed
2 tablespoons extra virgin olive
  oil, plus extra for brushing
5 basil sprigs
40g (1½oz/½ cup) finely grated
  Parmesan, plus extra to serve
½ tablespoon finely grated
  lemon zest
1 tablespoon freshly squeezed
  lemon juice
sea salt and cracked black pepper

FOR THE BASIL OIL

2 tablespoons extra virgin olive oil
1 basil sprig, leaves picked

TO SERVE

150g (5½oz) burrata, torn
a pinch of dried chilli
  (hot pepper) flakes
micro (baby) purple basil

Begin by making the flaxseed linguine. Put the flaxseed and half of the filtered water in a small bowl. Allow to sit for 5 minutes. Using a stick blender, give the mixture a quick blend to increase its glutinous effect. Mix the flour and salt together on a clean surface and make a well in the centre. Pour the flax mixture and the olive oil into the well and mix to form a dough. While mixing, add in the remaining filtered water, using less or more as necessary. Use a dough scraper to bring the ingredients the together and knead to a stiff, uniform dough. Form into a ball, then place in cling film (plastic wrap) and allow to rest for at least 30 minutes and up to 90 minutes.

Once the dough has rested, cut it into smaller pieces, roll each piece in flour and run it through a pasta machine, starting at the thickest setting and working your way down to the thinner ones. Stop at the second-to-last thinnest setting for the final press, then cut the pasta sheets into 3mm- (⅛in-) wide linguine strips using the relevant attachment on the machine. Spread over a baking paper-lined baking sheet and place in the freezer for 30 minutes.

Now make the asparagus pesto. Preheat a griddle pan over high heat. Brush the asparagus with olive oil and sprinkle with salt and pepper. Cook for 5–6 minutes or until just charred. Allow to cool slightly, then roughly chop. Place in a food processor with the olive oil, basil, Parmesan, lemon zest and juice, salt and pepper and process until smooth. Set aside.

To make the basil oil, grind the olive oil and basil together with a pestle and mortar. Transfer to a small bowl.

To cook the linguine, bring a large pot of salted water to a boil. Add the semi-frozen linguine to the boiling water, allow to return to a boil, then cook for 1–2 minutes. Once cooked, drain the pasta in a colander and return to the saucepan. Add the asparagus pesto to the linguine and stir to coat.

To serve, divide the linguine between 2 plates and top with the burrata, chilli flakes, basil oil, micro herbs and salt and pepper.

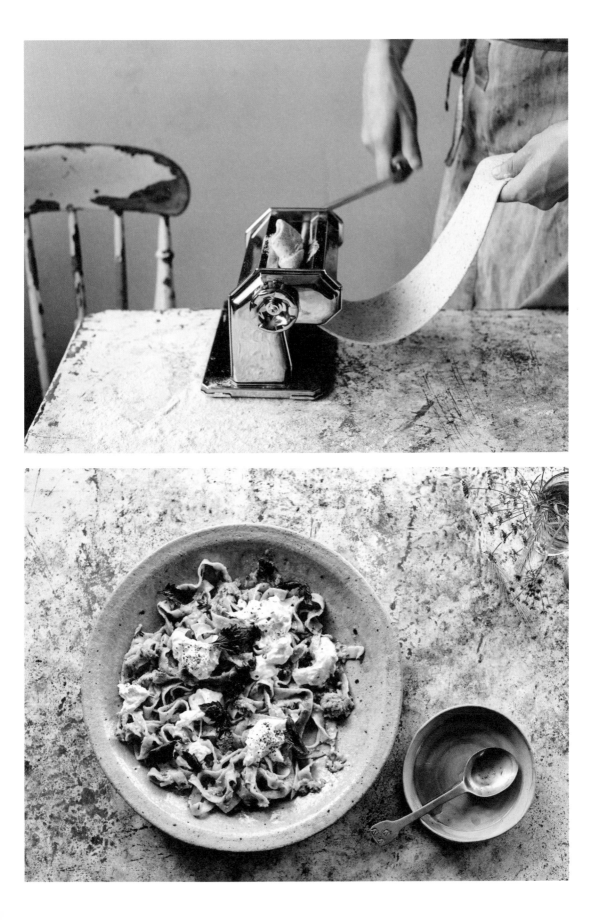

When humble sweet potato wedges start to get dull (I've done the sumac-sprinkled sweet potatoes to death!), you need to find ways of dressing them up and making them interesting again.

Looking for inspiration, I peered at the tubs of Thai red and green curry paste in the fridge (the ones that get used only once in a month, if that, and can live in your fridge for years!). I found myself wondering if I could use them as a way to spice up vegetables. So, I grabbed the red curry paste, loosened it with some olive oil and then coated some sweet potato wedges in the paste – the result is crazy-good! Especially when coupled with this basil raita.

SPRING GREEN SAAG CURRY
with spicy sweet potato wedges & basil raita (v)

SERVES 2–4

FOR THE SWEET POTATO WEDGES

3 tablespoons extra virgin olive oil
1 teaspoon Thai red curry paste
2 sweet potatoes

FOR THE SAAG CURRY

1 head of broccoli, florets and stem roughly chopped
150g (5½oz/heaped 1 cup) fresh or frozen peas
a small bunch coriander (cilantro), chopped (include the stalks)
4 handfuls baby spinach leaves
1 tablespoon grated ginger
1 green chilli (with seeds)
1 tablespoon cumin seeds, toasted
2 teaspoons ground turmeric
2 teaspoons garam masala
1 teaspoon sea salt
300ml (10½fl oz/1¼ cups) vegetable stock
2 tablespoons extra virgin olive oil
400ml (14fl oz) can full-fat coconut milk
½ head cauliflower, florets removed and trimmed
sea salt and cracked black pepper

Begin by roasting the sweet potato wedges. Preheat the oven to 200°C/400°F/Gas 6 and line a large baking sheet with baking paper.

Put the olive oil and red curry paste in a mixing bowl and whisk to combine and form a paste. Cut each sweet potato in half lengthways and then cut each half into 3–4 wedges depending on the size of the sweet potato. Add the sweet potato wedges to the mixing bowl with the red curry paste and toss to coat. Transfer the wedges to the baking sheet, laying them out in an even layer. Sprinkle with sea salt to taste and roast in the oven for 25 minutes or until golden brown and crisp. Remove from the oven. Set aside until ready to serve the curry.

To make the saag curry, place the broccoli, peas, coriander, baby spinach leaves, ginger, green chilli, cumin seeds, ground turmeric, garam masala and 1 teaspoon sea salt into a food processor. Blend the ingredients to a paste, then add the vegetable stock, 100ml (3½fl oz/scant ½ cup) at a time. Blend the ingredients a little more with each addition until the mixture is smooth.

INGREDIENTS & METHOD CONTINUE...

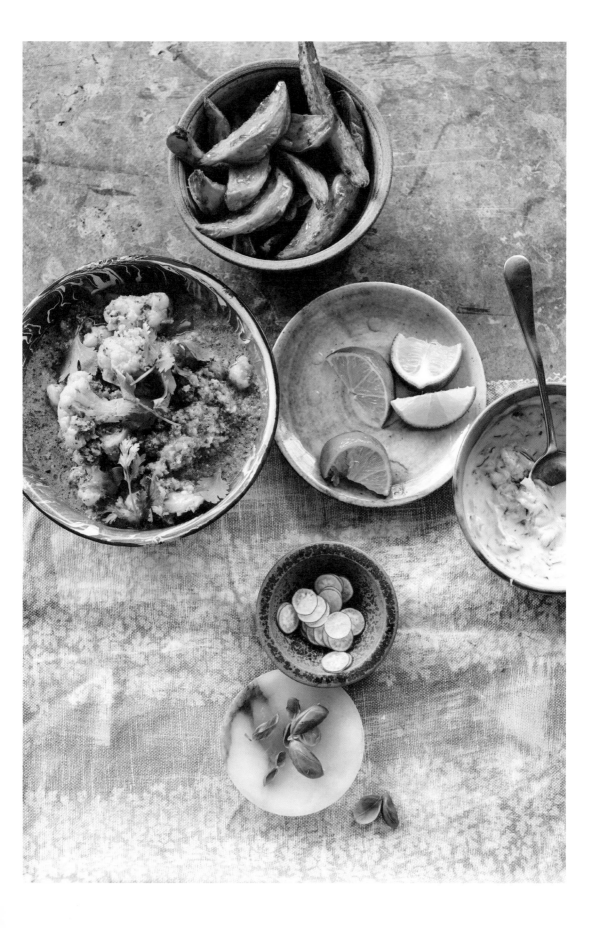

FOR THE BASIL RAITA

150g (5½oz/scant ⅔ cup)
   full-fat, natural yoghurt (vegan
   if necessary)
¼ cucumber, grated with skin on
finely grated zest and freshly
   squeezed juice of 1 lemon
a small handful basil leaves,
   finely sliced

TO GARNISH

1 lime, cut into quarters
2 radishes, thinly sliced
coriander (cilantro) leaves

Place a large, lidded sauté pan over a medium heat, add the olive oil, the saag mixture and the coconut milk, stir to combine and bring to the boil. Add the cauliflower florets to the saag, reduce the heat to low and cover the pan with the lid. Allow to simmer for 20 minutes or until the cauliflower is al dente.

While the saag is cooking, you can make the basil raita. In a small mixing bowl, place the yoghurt, grated cucumber, lemon zest and juice and sliced basil. Stir to combine. Season with sea salt and black pepper. Set aside.

Remove the lid from the pan and give the saag a gentle stir. Check to see if the cauliflower florets are just cooked. Now check for seasoning and add sea salt and black pepper to taste. Remove the pan from the heat and prepare to serve.

Spoon saag curry into the bottom of 4 shallow bowls, and then lay a few sweet potato wedges over the top of each bowl. Garnish with the basil raita, a lime wedge, radish slices and coriander leaves.

If you are usually compassionate, feel emotionally fulfilled, and enjoy loving deeply, you more than likely have a healthy heart chakra. You can easily maintain intimate relationships, but also have healthy personal boundaries. You are trusting, forgiving, non-judgmental, kind, and often radiate peace and calmness.

You have a strong connection with nature, you're reliable, people find themselves opening up to you, and you feel a sincere gratitude for everything that enters your life – even the challenging things. It is here that your energy begins to shift towards the spirit realm. Opening this chakra awakens you to the universal love surrounding and filling you.

RICOTTA, COURGETTE & PARMESAN FRITTERS
with salsa verde

SERVES 2

FOR THE FRITTERS

1 tablespoon ground flaxseed
80g (2¾oz/scant ⅓ cup) firm ricotta cheese
1 courgette (zucchini), about 220g/7¾oz, washed and grated
1 teaspoon finely grated lemon zest
40g (1½oz/½ cup) finely grated Parmesan cheese, plus extra to serve
50g (1¾oz/½ cup) quinoa flakes or breadcrumbs
1 tablespoon extra virgin olive oil, plus extra for greasing
sea salt and cracked black pepper

FOR THE SALSA VERDE

6 flat-leaf parsley sprigs, leaves picked
6 basil sprigs, leaves picked
4 mint sprigs, leaves picked
freshly squeezed juice of 1 lemon
cracked black pepper
100ml (3½fl oz/scant ½ cup) extra virgin olive oil
½ teaspoon sea salt

Put the ground flaxseed in a small bowl with 2 tablespoons water and whisk to combine. Set aside while you make the salsa verde.

To make the salsa verde, put the herbs and lemon juice in a food processor and blitz until you have a thin paste. Trickle the olive oil into the processor until you have a thin pesto. Season to taste and set aside.

Using a stick blender, give the flaxseed mixture a quick blend to increase its glutinous effect, which will help the fritters bind together. Place it, along with the ricotta, grated courgette, lemon rind, Parmesan and quinoa flakes or breadcrumbs, in a medium mixing bowl. Season with salt and pepper and stir to combine. Allow the mixture to sit for 15 minutes.

Heat a little oil in a large non-stick frying pan over a high heat. Working in batches, cook tablespoons of the mixture for 2–3 minutes on each side or until golden.

Serve the fritters with a drizzle of salsa verde and some extra Parmesan over the top.

For anyone who isn't familar with Buddha bowls – they are bowls of delicious food which are packed so full that they have a rounded 'belly' appearance on top, much like the belly of a Buddha. And they make fabulous meals!

They offer a chance to nourish your body with a plethora of your favourite foods and flavours that you may not have otherwise put together. The key is to create a base and dressing that complement the rest of the ingredients.

KIMCHI-MARINATED KALE BUDDHA BOWL
with black rice pilaf (v)

SERVES 2

FOR THE BLACK RICE PILAF

150g (5½oz/scant 1 cup)
    black rice
2 tablespoons extra virgin olive oil
½ teaspoon sea salt
2 celery sticks, washed, trimmed
    and thinly sliced
6 radishes, washed, trimmed and
    thinly sliced into rounds
seeds from ¼ large pomegranate
3 tablespoons raw pistachios,
    roughly chopped

FOR THE KIMCHI-
MARINATED KALE

2 tablespoons kimchi (make sure
    it is vegan)
2 tablespoons toasted sesame oil
1 tablespoon freshly squeezed
    lime juice
1 tablespoon extra virgin olive oil
80g (2¾oz) curly kale, washed
    and leaves roughly torn
    off the stem

FOR THE BUDDHA BOWL

8 roasted sweet potato wedges
8–10 blanched broccoli florets
4 tablespoons edamame beans
flesh of 1 avocado, peeled, pitted
    and sliced
1 tablespoon pickled ginger
white sesame seeds
2 wedges of lime

Begin by making the pilaf. Put the rice in a saucepan and cover with 600ml (21fl oz/2½ cups) water. Place the saucepan over a medium–high heat and cook uncovered for 35 minutes or until the water has been completely absorbed and the rice is cooked through. Add a little more water to the pan if needed. Rinse the cooked rice through a fine colander to remove the black residue. Allow to drip dry in the colander while you prepare the rest of the ingredients.

For the kimchi-marinated kale, place the kimchi, sesame oil, lime juice and olive oil in a food processor and process until smooth. Add a few tablespoons of water if needed to loosen the dressing. Massage half the dressing into the kale leaves for 2 minutes, or until the kale is wilted and soft from the dressing acids. Set aside the rest of the dressing and the kale while you finish off the rice pilaf.

Put the cooked black rice in a mixing bowl, add the olive oil and sea salt and toss to combine. Add the celery, radishes, pomegranate seeds and pistachios. Toss to combine again.

Divide the kale between 2 large shallow serving bowls, then divide the rice into the bowls, too. Fill the rest of the bowls with roasted sweet potato wedges, blanched broccoli florets, edamame beans, avocado slices, pickled ginger, white sesame seeds and wedges of lime. Serve with the remaining dressing drizzled over the top and enjoy immediately.

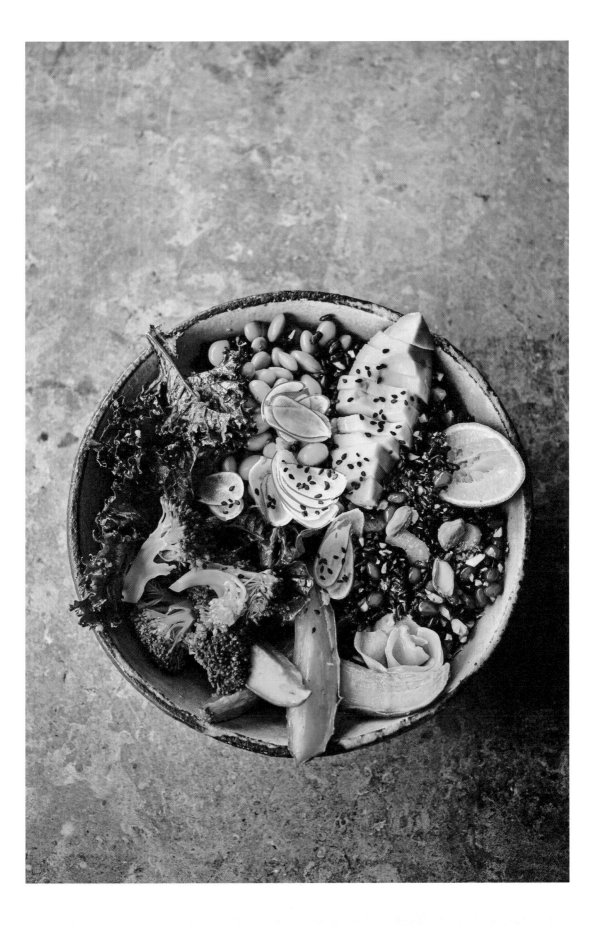

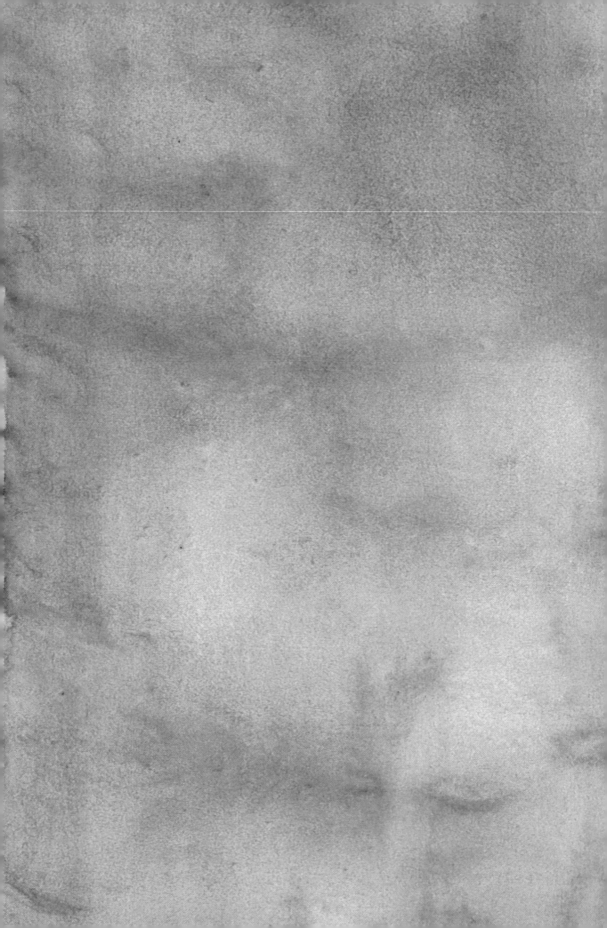

THROAT CHAKRA
truth

Key foods for the throat chakra:
BLUE FOOD: blueberry, raisin, cranberry,
goji berry, plum, rhubarb
HERBS TO HELP THE THROAT AND THYROID: sage,
elderberry, echinacea, manuka honey, ginger
VITAMIN-C-RICH FOOD:
strawberry, parsley, goji berry
IODINE-RICH FOOD:
kelp, sunflower seeds
Avoid stimulating foods, such as caffeine
and refined sugars

Buying a plain kombucha and adding your own flavour twist is a great way to make kombucha a little more interesting and a little more tailored to your palate. I generally buy the ginger-flavoured kombucha and then add fruits and herbs to it. Basil is a good herb to use as it works with so many fruits such as strawberries, raspberries and blueberries – as in this recipe for the throat chakra.

Just make sure you don't blend the ingredients together in the blender because you'll end up with a big, fizzy mess! But if you don't have a pestle and mortar you can blend the fruit and herbs together in the blender and then add it all to the kombucha.

POACHED PEAR & RHUBARB COMPOTE & PISTACHIO CRUMBLE
with blueberry & basil kombucha (v)

SERVES 2

FOR THE POACHED PEAR
& RHUBARB COMPOTE

2 large or 3 medium pears,
   cut into quarters and cored
2 rhubarb stalks, chopped into
   4cm (1½in) lengths
200ml (7fl oz/generous ¾ cup)
   freshly squeezed orange juice
3 cardamom pods
1 cinnamon stick
1 star anise
2 tablespoons yoghurt (vegan if
   necessary) or leftover labneh

FOR THE BLUEBERRY &
BASIL KOMBUCHA

50g (1¾oz/scant ½ cup)
   blueberries
3 basil sprigs, leaves picked
700ml (24fl oz/scant 3 cups)
   plain, store-bought kombucha

FOR THE PISTACHIO
CRUMBLE

50g (1¾oz/⅓ cup) raw
   pistachios, roughly chopped
20g (⅔oz/scant ¼ cup) dried
   goji berries
1 tablespoon chia seeds

Begin by making the poached pear and rhubarb compote. Preheat the oven to 200°C/400°F/Gas 6. Line a roasting tray with baking paper.

Combine all the compote ingredients (except the yoghurt or labneh) in the roasting tray and cover with kitchen foil. Bake in the preheated oven for 10 minutes, then remove the foil and bake for a further 10 minutes. (If your pears are particularly hard and unripe, you may want to bake them for an extra 10 minutes before adding the rhubarb.) Remove the roasting tray from the oven and allow to cool while you make the kombucha.

Place the blueberries and basil leaves in a pestle and mortar. Muddle together until you create a paste and the basil leaves have been incorporated with the blueberries. Now add to a jug large enough to hold up to 1 litre (35fl oz/4 cups) of liquid. Pour in the kombucha and stir to combine. Allow to infuse for 10–20 minutes.

Combine the pistachio crumble ingredients in a small mixing bowl. Set aside.

To serve, place the compote into 2 breakfast bowls, top with a dollop of yoghurt or labneh and then sprinkle with the pistachio crumble. Enjoy with the blueberry and basil kombucha.

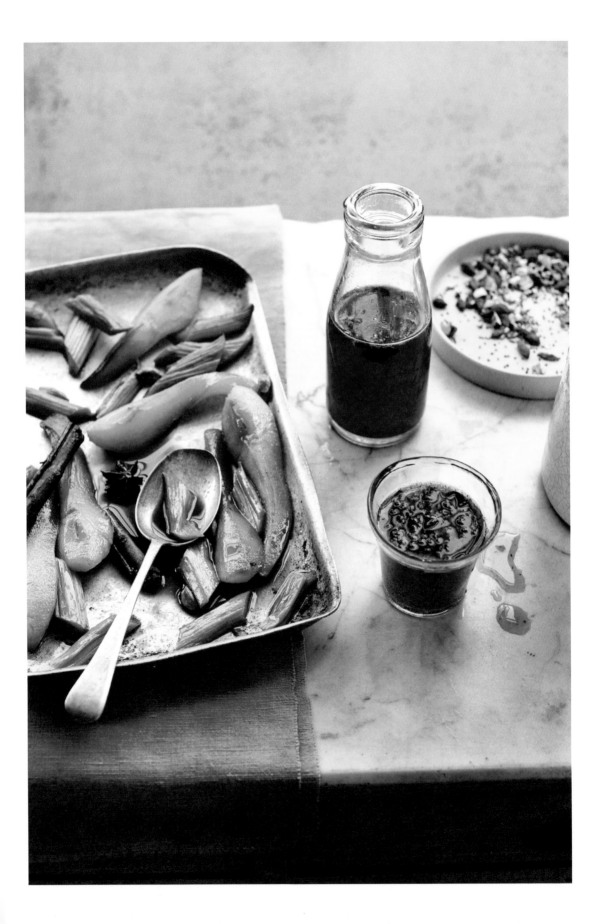

This porridge is the perfect blend of soft, sweet, stewed fruit and hearty, filling porridge. The result, I must say, is stellar!

Once you've made the porridge, you'll keep coming back to it, time and time again, experimenting with other fruit, spice and grain combinations.

Pears make an easy substitution for the apples and, to stay true to the throat chakra, you could substitute the blackberries for blackcurrants or plums.

BLACKBERRY, BUCKWHEAT & STEWED APPLE PORRIDGE (v)

SERVES 2

3 eating apples, peeled, cored and roughly chopped into wedges
80g (2¾oz/½ cup) buckwheat groats or (1 cup) rolled oats
360ml (12fl oz/1½ cups) filtered water
1 teaspoon ground cinnamon
100ml (3½fl oz/scant ½ cup) oat milk or milk of your choice (optional)
200g (7oz/1½ cups) fresh or frozen blackberries
coconut yoghurt, to serve
toasted almonds, roughly chopped, to serve

Put the apples, buckwheat groats, water and cinnamon into a large heavy-based saucepan. Stir to combine and place over a medium heat. Cover the saucepan with a lid and bring the mixture to a gentle simmer, stirring every 4–5 minutes to make sure the buckwheat groats don't stick to the bottom on the pan.

Allow to cook for a further 10–20 minutes or until the apples are tender, the buckwheat groats have softened and everything is nicely cooked and combined.

Remove from the heat and add the milk to loosen the mixture if desired. Add the blackberries. Stir through and serve immediately topped with some yoghurt and toasted almonds.

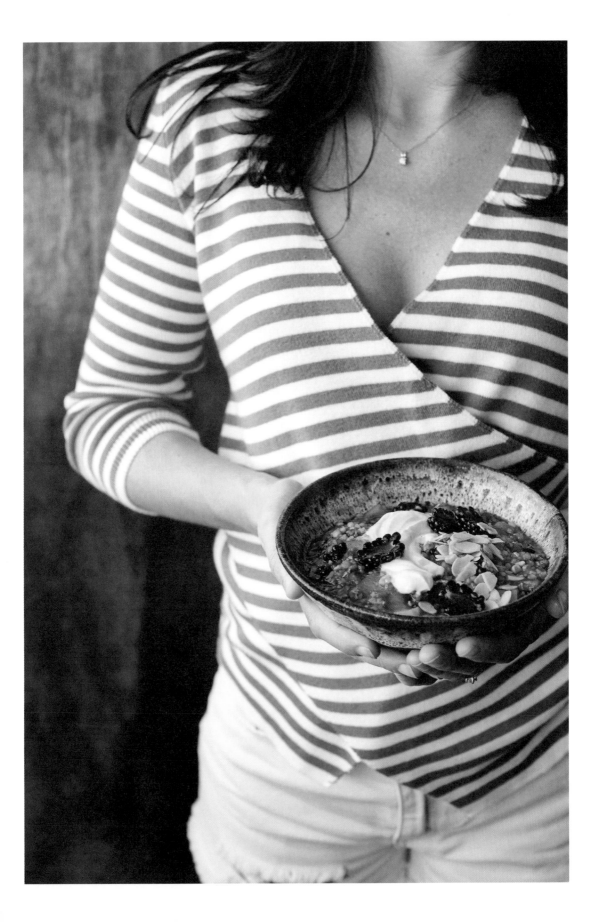

During the years I worked as a chalet chef in the French Alps, I served traditional French toast to the guests on Christmas morning and it's become a bit of a tradition in my family now, too. This is my vegan version, which uses ground chia seeds to thicken the batter.

I have switched regular sliced bread for raisin bread as I think the warming cinnamon flavour of the raisin bread complements the caramelized bananas really well.

RAISIN BREAD FRENCH TOAST
with a warming ginger latte (v)

SERVES 2

FOR THE FRENCH TOAST

1 tablespoon chia seeds
200ml (7fl oz/generous ¾ cup) oat milk or milk of your choice
1 teaspoon vanilla extract
½ teaspoon ground cinnamon
1 tablespoon maple syrup, plus extra to serve
1 tablespoon coconut oil, for frying
4–6 thick slices of raisin bread
full-fat, natural Greek yoghurt (vegan if necessary), to serve

FOR THE CARAMELIZED BANANAS

2 tablespoons maple syrup
2 tablespoons coconut sugar
1 tablespoon coconut oil
1 banana, peeled and chopped into slices

FOR THE GINGER LATTE

60g (2oz/½ cup) cashews
400ml (14fl oz/1¾ cups) oat milk or milk of your choice
120ml (4fl oz/½ cup) coconut milk
2–4 pitted dates
1 teaspoon ground cinnamon, plus extra to serve (optional)
½ teaspoon ground cardamom
¼ teaspoon ground cloves
½ teaspoon ground ginger
1 teaspoon vanilla extract

Begin by grinding the chia seeds into a fine powder using a NutriBullet or a food processor. (This isn't essential, but the finished French toast will look more refined if using a powder.)

Whisk the chia seeds, milk, vanilla, cinnamon and maple syrup together in a large bowl and refrigerate for 10–20 minutes. This will give the chia seeds time to thicken the mixture and give it an 'eggy' texture.

Heat the coconut oil in a large frying pan over a medium–high heat. Dip each slice of raisin bread into the chia mixture, allowing the bread to sit in the mixture for 20 seconds or so on each side. Fry the bread for 3–4 minutes on each side until golden brown.

To make the caramelized bananas, place another non-stick frying pan over a medium heat. Add the maple syrup, coconut sugar and oil to the pan and stir to combine until the sugar has dissolved. Add the banana and coat in the caramel, then allow to bubble away for around 3–4 minutes until the banana is soft. Remove from the heat. Serve the caramelized bananas over the French toast. Drizzle the remaining sauce from the caramelized bananas over the top. Serve with a dollop of yoghurt and a little extra maple syrup if desired.

To make the warming ginger latte, add all the ingredients to a blender and blend until creamy and smooth. Pour the mixture into a small saucepan and heat on low–medium heat until warmed through. Pour into mugs and sprinkle with some cinnamon powder if desired. Enjoy alongside the French toast.

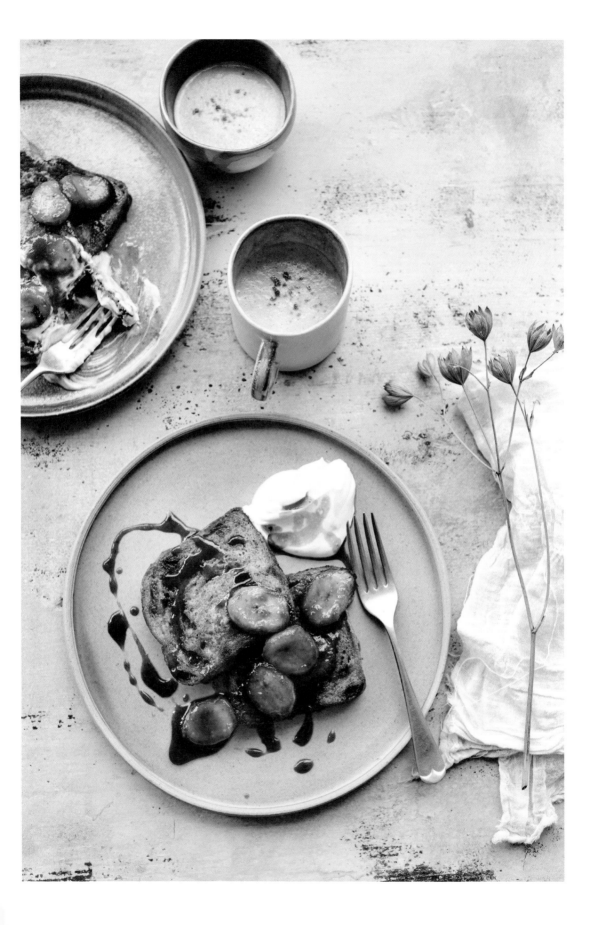

Part savoury crêpe, part flatbread, a socca is both simple and delicious. Socca is traditionally made from just chickpea flour, water and olive oil (with some cracked black pepper), baked on a large round pan in a wood-fired oven, then rustically scraped off the pan into large slabs and served while still warm. It has a custardy interior and is golden on top and crispy around the edges.

As usual, I've taken some liberties with tradition and put my own twist on a basic recipe. I decided to throw in some extra flavour with the asparagus and goat's cheese to add another dimension to the dish.

This is an any-time-of-day kind of recipe and is extremely versatile, so feel free to add spinach, pesto, feta and other vegetables into your socca to add variety and flavour to this easy-to-prepare meal.

ASPARAGUS & GOAT'S CURD SOCCA

SERVES 2

120g (4oz/1 cup) chickpea (gram) flour
240ml (8fl oz/1 cup) water
½ teaspoon sea salt, plus extra to top
2 teaspoons lemon juice
¼ teaspoon bicarbonate of soda (baking soda)
2 tablespoons extra virgin olive oil
6 asparagus spears, washed and trimmed
3 tablespoons goat's curd, roughly crumbled
cracked black pepper
Parmesan shavings, to serve
baby spinach leaves, to serve

Place the chickpea flour and salt in a medium mixing bowl and slowly whisk in the water and the lemon juice. Cover and allow the batter to rest for a few hours, or preferably overnight.

When ready to make the socca, preheat the oven to 230°C/450°F/Gas 8. Measure 1 tablespoon of the olive oil into a cast-iron skillet and place in the oven to preheat.

Whisk the bicarbonate of soda and the remaining olive oil into the socca batter until smooth.

Remove the preheated skillet from the oven and pour the batter in. Scatter the asparagus spears and goat's curd over the batter and then top with a few grinds of black pepper and a pinch of sea salt.

Bake in the preheated oven for 20 minutes, or until the socca is set and golden around the edges.

Remove from oven and sprinkle with Parmesan shavings and baby spinach leaves.

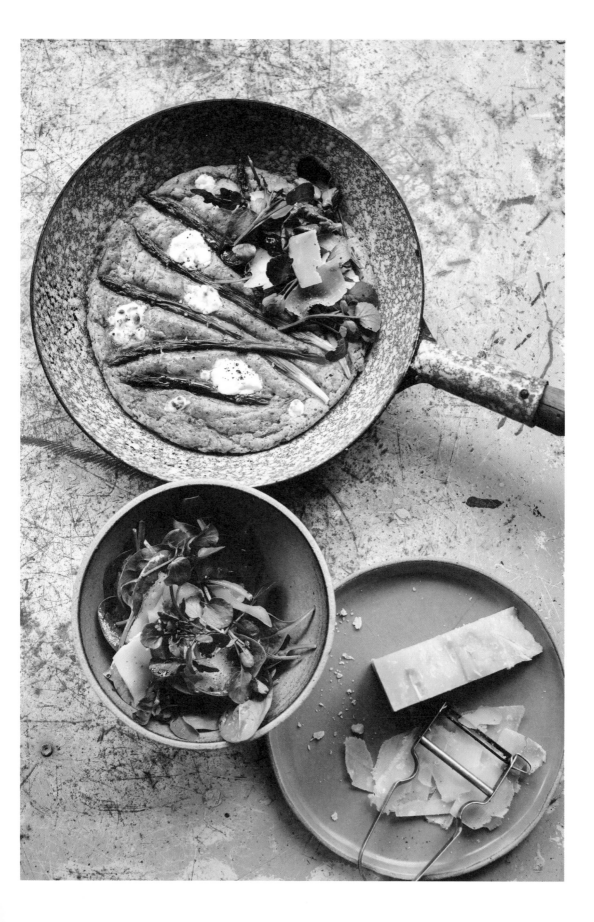

I like to imagine a galette being invented by a lazy pastry chef who couldn't be bothered with all the fuss and perfection pastry work often demands. I personally love rustic pastry and this nutty spelt pastry is so easy to whip up. Keep a batch in the freezer and this galette can be ready in minimal time and with very little effort on your part.

BEETROOT, SPINACH & GOAT'S CHEESE GALETTE

SERVES 4

FOR THE PASTRY

100g (3½oz/¾ cup) spelt flour
100g (3½oz/¾ cup) wholemeal (wholegrain) flour
1 teaspoon baking powder
½ teaspoon salt
120ml (4fl oz/½ cup) water
120ml (4fl oz/½ cup) extra virgin olive oil

FOR THE GALETTE FILLING

5 beetroot (beets), about 450g (1lb) total weight
2 handfuls baby spinach leaves
1 teaspoon freshly squeezed lemon juice
1 teaspoon extra virgin olive oil
a pinch of sea salt
1 tablespoon goat's cheese
1 teaspoon ground almonds
1 tablespoon thyme leaves

FOR THE DRESSED LEAVES

1 handful beetroot (beet) greens
1 handful baby spinach leaves
1 teaspoon extra virgin olive oil
½ teaspoon wholegrain mustard
1 teaspoon balsamic vinegar

TO SERVE

2 tablespoons goat's cheese
1 tablespoon sunflower seeds

Preheat the oven to 180°C/350°F/Gas 4 and begin by making the pastry. Sift the flours, baking powder and salt into a large mixing bowl. Pour the water and olive oil into the flour and combine using a wooden spoon or your hands until a dough is formed. Remove the dough from the bowl and place it onto a large sheet of baking paper. Using a rolling pin, roll the dough into a 30–35cm (12–14in) round disk that is roughly 2–3mm (⅛in) thick. Trim the edges if desired.

To make the filling, put the beetroot into a steamer basket set over a pan of water and cook over a medium heat for 25 minutes. Once cooked through, remove from the steamer and allow to cool. Once cooled, remove the beetroot skins and slice into 2mm (⅛in) thick slices.

Put the spinach in a small saucepan, add the lemon juice, olive oil and a pinch of sea salt and turn the heat to medium. Cook for 30 seconds –1 minute until just wilted, allow to cool slightly then remove from pan. Squeeze the spinach to remove excess water.

Using a palette knife, spread the goat's cheese thinly over the pastry, stopping 2cm (¾in) from the edge. Sprinkle the ground almonds over, then the spinach and then the beetroot slices, finishing with the thyme leaves and always leaving the 2cm (¾in) border at the edge. Fold the bare edges of the pastry over the filling. Slide the galette onto a baking sheet and bake for 35–45 minutes, or until the pastry is cooked and golden. Meanwhile, combine the beetroot leaves (tear up the big ones), spinach, olive oil, mustard and balsamic vinegar in a bowl. Toss to combine.

Once cooked, remove the galette from the oven and scatter over some goat's cheese and sunflower seeds. Serve with the dressed leaves.

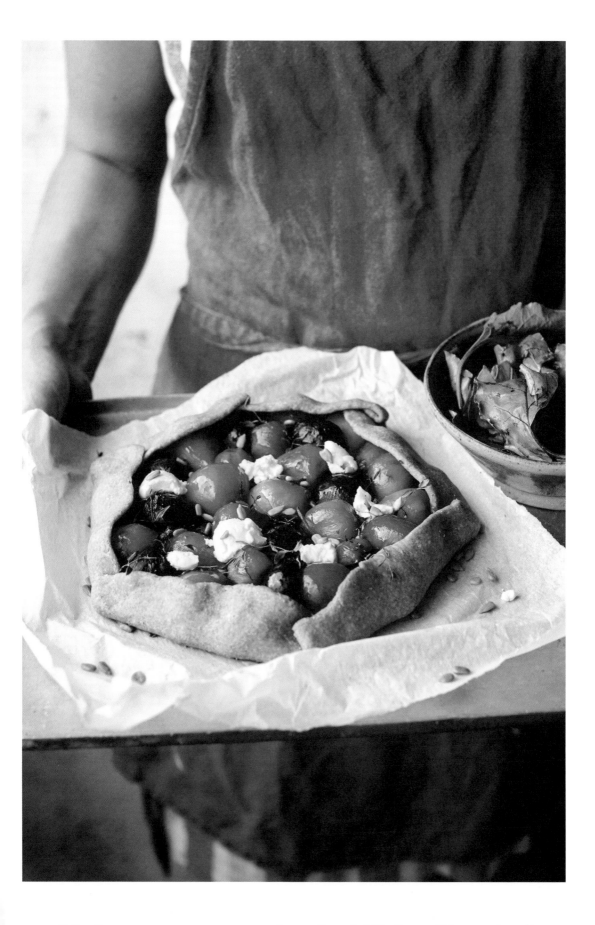

Chickpea 'tofu' was such an exciting recipe find when I heard about it. I immediately tried it out in all forms and haven't stopped whipping up batches of it since. Not only does it taste better than real tofu, but it's cheap to make and so easy to prepare. The almond crumb that coats the chips is full of flavour and creates a lovely crispness for these healthy and tasty chips.

CHICKPEA 'TOFU' CHIPS
with tomato sauce (v)

SERVES 2–4

FOR THE TOMATO SAUCE

1 tablespoon extra virgin olive oil
1 celery stick, finely diced
½ teaspoon chopped thyme
   leaves
1 bay leaf
1 x 400g (14oz) can of plum
   tomatoes, or 450g (1lb) fresh
   plum tomatoes if in season
1 tablespoon tomato purée (paste)
1 tablespoon apple cider vinegar
1 tablespoon date syrup
3–4 basil sprigs, leaves picked
sea salt and cracked black pepper

FOR THE CHICKPEA
'TOFU' CHIPS

coconut oil, for greasing
150g (5½oz/heaped 1 cup)
   chickpea (gram) flour
1 teaspoon fine sea salt
a pinch of ground turmeric

FOR THE ALMOND CRUMB

120g (4¼oz/scant 1 cup) whole
   blanched or (1¼ cups) ground
   almonds
2 teaspoons sweet smoked
   paprika
1 tablespoon dried oregano
1 teaspoon fine sea salt
20g (⅔oz/2¼ tablespoons)
   buckwheat or chickpea
   (gram) flour

For the tomato sauce, heat the olive oil in a wide saucepan and sweat the celery, thyme and bay leaf. Once soft, add the tomatoes, tomato purée and apple cider vinegar. Stir well, then add the date syrup. Reduce to a simmer over a low heat. Add the basil stalks and simmer for 20–30 minutes. Season to taste, then blend until smooth and pass through a fine sieve, if desired. Cool and pour into a container and refrigerate for now.

To make the chickpea 'tofu', grease a 15cm (6in) square baking pan with coconut oil. Put the chickpea flour in a bowl with the salt and turmeric. Now, slowly add 360ml (12fl oz/1½ cups) water, whisking to combine the whole time. Put another 360ml (12fl oz/1½ cups) water into a saucepan and bring to the boil. Reduce the heat to a very low simmer, then add the chickpea flour mixture, beating vigorously for 5–6 minutes until thick, smooth and glossy. Immediately pour into the prepared baking pan and cool at room temperature for about 45 minutes.

Meanwhile, for the almond crumb, put the almonds, paprika, oregano and salt into a food processor and pulse until the almonds are fine (you may have to scrape the sides between pulses). If you are using ground almonds, simply combine all the ingredients in a bowl. Tip the crumb into a wide shallow bowl and set aside. Preheat the oven to 200°C/400°F/Gas 6 and line a baking sheet with baking paper.

Turn out the chickpea 'tofu' onto a board and cut into sticks. Then whisk 3–4 tablespoons water, little by little, into the buckwheat or chickpea flour to create a smooth loose batter. One by one, submerge the sticks in the batter, then dip into the almond crumb to fully coat and place on the prepared baking sheet. Bake for 20 minutes, or until hot and crispy. Serve with the chilled tomato sauce for dipping. The cooked crumbed tofu will keep up to 3 days stored in an airtight container in the fridge.

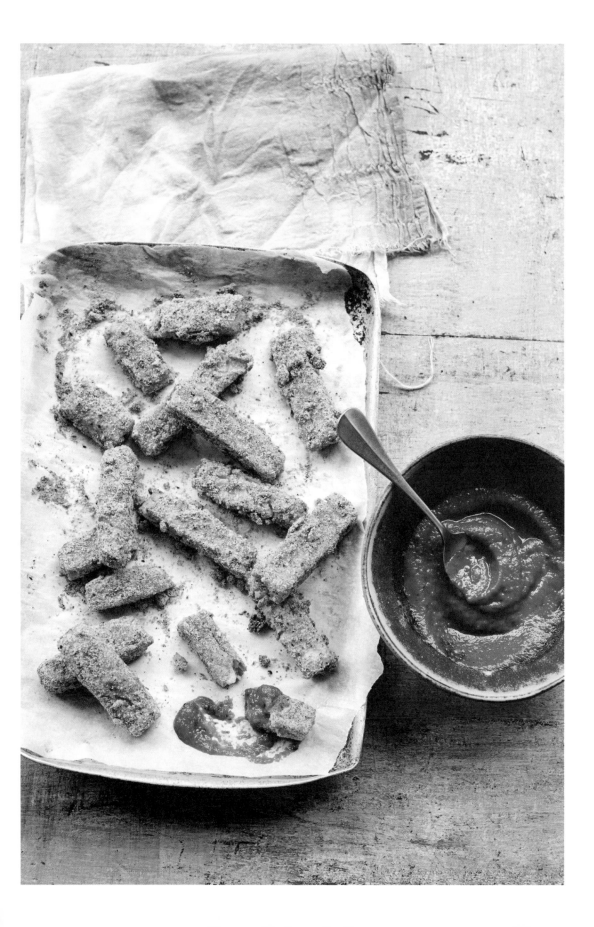

I called this throat chakra chapter 'truth' because so much of your authentic self-expression is tied up in your ability to speak your truth. Great conversations and creativity are cornerstones of a healthy throat chakra, as is the ability to be a good listener. These are traits that make for a happy and fulfilling life, so ensure you can express yourself through all forms of communication.

HORSERADISH, WATERCRESS, CELERIAC & APPLE SALAD
served with sundried tomato & basil cheese spread (v)

SERVES 2

25g (1oz/¼ cup) raw walnuts
2 small Granny Smith apples
juice of 1 lemon
½ small celeriac (celery root)
1 fennel bulb, trimmed and halved
2 handfuls watercress
crisp breads or crackers, to serve

FOR THE 'CHEESE' SPREAD

40g (1½oz/⅓ cup) raw cashews
2 tablespoons nutritional
    yeast flakes
¼ teaspoon sea salt
100ml (3½fl oz/scant ½ cup)
    unsweetened almond milk or
    milk of your choice
½ tablespoon tomato
    purée (paste)
1 tablespoon extra virgin olive oil
1 tablespoon agar flakes
2 tablespoons sundried tomatoes
    in oil, finely chopped
1 tablespoon basil leaves,
    finely chopped

FOR THE DRESSING

100ml (3½fl oz/scant ½ cup)
    coconut yoghurt
2 tablespoons extra virgin olive oil
½ teaspoon Dijon mustard
½ tablespoon finely chopped
    parsley
½ teaspoon hot horseradish paste
sea salt and cracked black pepper

Begin by making the 'cheese' spread. Place the cashews, nutritional yeast and salt in a food processor and blend until a fine crumb forms. In a small saucepan, whisk together the milk, tomato purée and olive oil. Place the saucepan over a medium heat, then sprinkle in the agar flakes and stir to combine. Remove from the heat and allow to sit for 5 minutes. Return the pan to a high heat and bring to the boil, continuously and vigorously whisking. Now reduce to a simmer and, using a silicon spatula, stir occasionally over a low heat for 5 minutes. Remove the pan from the heat and quickly pour the mixture into a food processor. Add the sundried tomatoes and basil and process until smooth. The mixture should be very thick. Line a ramekin or mould with cling film (plastic wrap) and press the cheese spread into the ramekin. Refrigerate to set for 1–2 hours.

Preheat the oven to 150°C/300°F/Gas 2. Place the walnuts on a baking sheet and roast for 15 minutes or until lightly golden. Remove from the oven and set aside to cool a little before roughly chopping.

Core, quarter and julienne the apples into matchsticks. Toss with the lemon juice in a large mixing bowl. Peel the celeriac and julienne the celeriac, too. Immediately add to the apple slices and toss. Thinly shave the fennel bulb and add this, too.

Whisk together all the ingredients for the dressing and season with salt and pepper. Add to the salad and combine gently.

Scatter the watercress leaves over 2 plates. Divide the salad over the watercress and sprinkle with the chopped walnuts. Serve with crisp breads or crackers and the cheese spread.

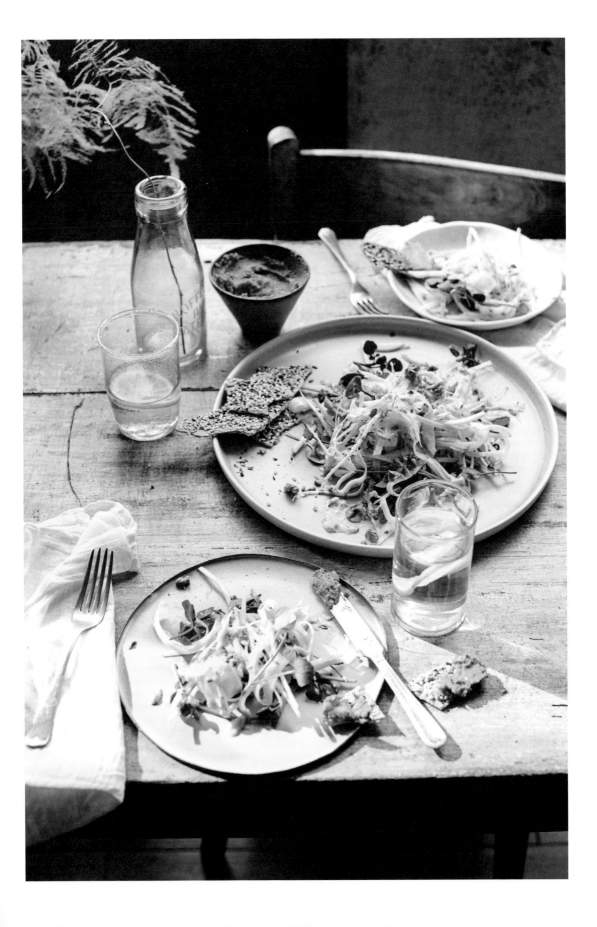

In this dish I have skewered the chickpea tofu from the recipe earlier in this chapter (page 132) and lightly grilled it to add some smokiness to the chickpea flavour. This salad is also a good dish to have all on its own and can make a great lunchtime salad.

GREEN BEAN & ARTICHOKE QUINOA SALAD
with grilled chickpea tofu skewers & pomegranate jus (v)

SERVES 2

½ recipe quantity Chickpea 'Tofu' without the crumb (see page 132)
2 tablespoons flaked (slivered) almonds, toasted, to serve

FOR THE SALAD

100g (3½oz/1 cup) sundried tomatoes in oil
1 teaspoon ground cumin
200g (7oz/heaped 1 cup) cooked quinoa
100g (3½oz) green (French) beans, trimmed and blanched
2 preserved artichokes in oil, drained and cut into wedges
40g (1½oz/⅓ cup) kalamata olives, pitted
1 handful rocket (arugula) leaves

FOR THE POMEGRANATE JUS

¼ pomegranate
1 tablespoon coconut yoghurt
1 teaspoon pomegranate molasses
sea salt and cracked black pepper

For the salad, put the sundried tomatoes, including their oil, and the cumin in a food processor and process to a smooth paste.

Put the paste in a mixing bowl, add the cooked quinoa and stir to completely coat the quinoa. Add the blanched green beans, drained artichokes, kalamata olives and rocket leaves and toss to combine. Set aside.

To make the pomegranate jus, hold the pomegranate over a bowl and carefully remove half the seeds. Set aside.

Over another small mixing bowl, squeeze the remaining pomegranate seeds from the shell and allow the juice to collect in the bowl. Discard the shell and remove any white pith that falls into the bowl. Add the remaining jus ingredients, except the seasoning, and whisk to combine. Season to taste.

To cook the chickpea tofu skewers, cut the chickpea tofu into 4 batons and thread onto 4 skewers. Heat a griddle pan over a high heat. Brush the tofu and pan with a little olive oil and cook the chickpea tofu skewers for a few minutes on each side until golden brown.

To serve, divide the salad between 2 plates, then top with the chickpea tofu skewers, drizzle with pomegranate jus and sprinkle over the toasted almonds and reserved pomegranate seeds.

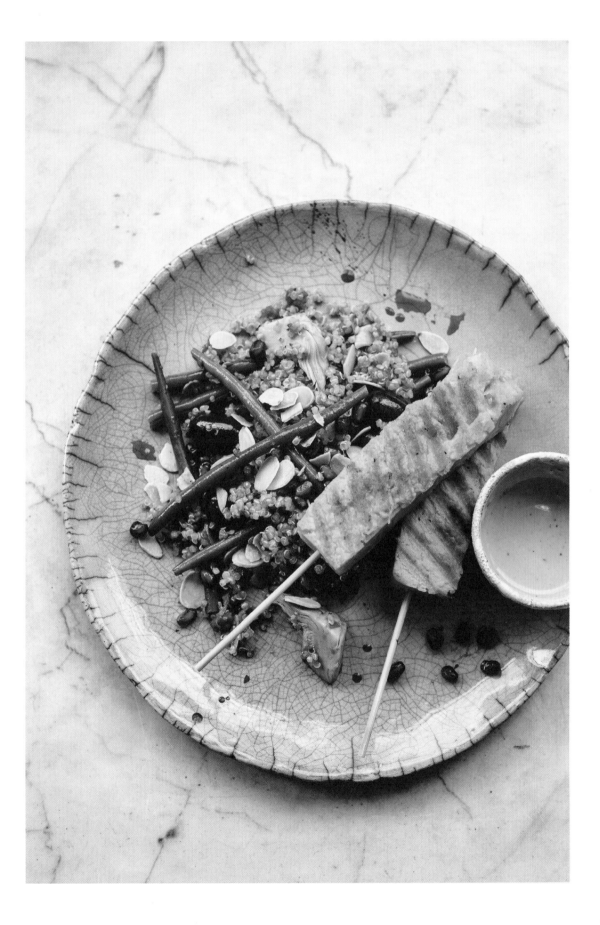

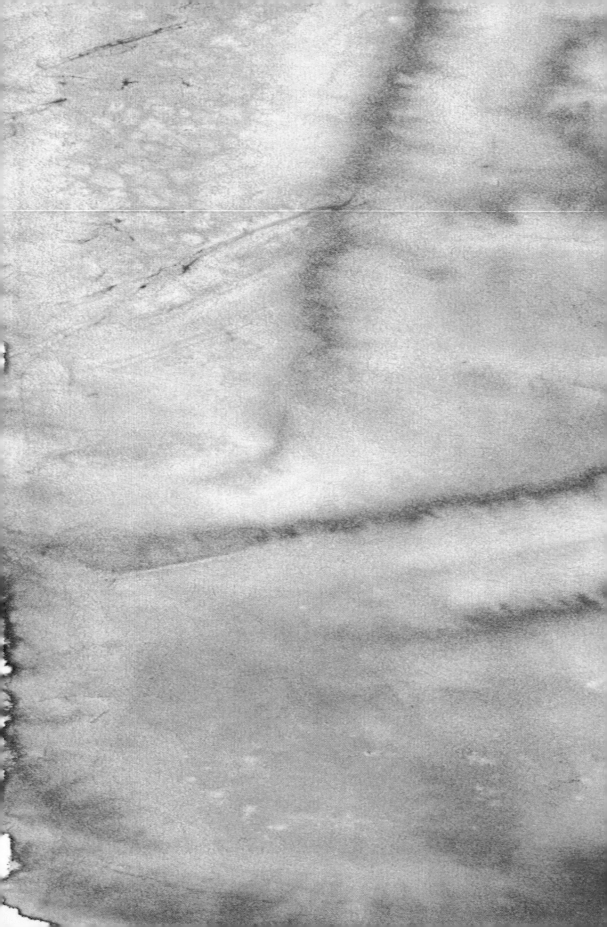

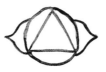

THIRD-EYE CHAKRA

intuition

Key foods for the third-eye chakra:
PURPLE FOOD: blackberry, red cabbage, grape,
radicchio, balsamic vinegar, fig, olive
STIMULATING FOOD: matcha, cacao
CALMING FOOD: chamomile, lemon verbena

This may seem totally self-indulgent and just a reason to eat chocolate at breakfast, but to be honest it's the perfect time of the day for chocolate – or rather its source, raw cacao. The caffeine in cacao gives you a natural high and having caffeine at this time of day won't disrupt your sleep patterns. It helps to boost your energy for the day ahead, so jump right into this porridge knowing your chocolate cravings will be satisfied and your circadian rhythm healthily maintained.

HAZELNUT & CACAO PORRIDGE
with almond butter (v)

SERVES 2

FOR THE PORRIDGE

110g (3¾oz/heaped 1 cup) rolled oats
a pinch of sea salt
1 tablespoon raw cacao powder
1 tablespoon vanilla extract
440ml (15½fl oz/scant 2 cups) oat milk, or milk of your choice, plus a drop more if needed
2 tablespoons maple syrup or date syrup (optional)

TO SERVE

almond butter
roasted hazelnuts, roughly chopped
cacao nibs (optional)

Combine all the ingredients for the porridge in a small saucepan. Place over a low–medium heat and stir to combine. Slowly bring the porridge to a steady simmer while stirring occasionally. Once the oats are cooked and tender, remove from the heat and add a little more oat milk if desired.

Divide the porridge into 2 breakfast bowls and serve with a dollop of almond butter, and a sprinkling of chopped roasted hazelnuts. Top with cacao nibs for an extra caffeine hit, if desired.

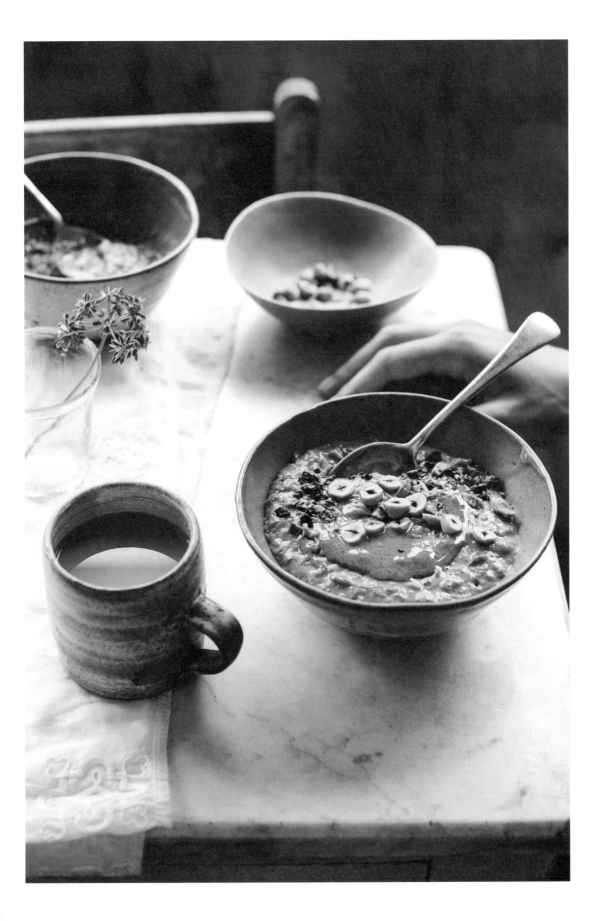

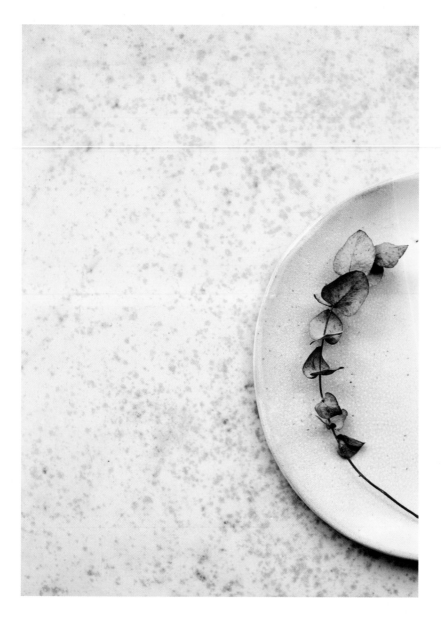

TO BALANCE YOUR THIRD-EYE CHAKRA IT CAN BE A
GOOD PRACTICE TO START KEEPING A DREAM JOURNAL
AS A WAY OF TAPPING INTO YOUR UNCONSCIOUS MIND.
I ALSO FIND STAR GAZING A LOVELY WAY TO OPEN
UP YOUR THIRD-EYE CHAKRA, AS STARING INTO THE
UNIVERSE THAT EXISTS AROUND US CAN OPEN OUR
MINDS TO THE MUCH LARGER PICTURE WE LIVE IN.

Cacao nibs are high in an alkaloid compound called theobromine. It's a nervous system stimulant resembling caffeine in its physiological effects that dilates the blood vessels, therefore creating a stimulating effect for our minds in much the same way that caffeine does. This effect is often welcome in the morning when we need to add a little more fire to our energy centres. This granola is the perfect pick-me-up – the bitterness of the cacao nibs is balanced by the sweetness of the coconut and the addition of the walnuts make this a symphony of nutty, bitter chocolate and sweet coconut happiness!

Enjoy with a creamy kefir or nut milk of your choice; I love cashew milk here.

PICK-ME-UP CACAO GRANOLA (v)

SERVES 8

150g (5½oz/1½ cups) rolled oats
50g (1¾oz/⅔ cup) desiccated (dried shredded) coconut
75g (2½oz/scant ½ cup) walnuts, roughly chopped
25g (1oz/3 tablespoons) cacao nibs
1 teaspoon ground cinnamon
2 teaspoons vanilla extract
5 tablespoons maple syrup
40g (1½oz/3 tablespoons) coconut oil

Preheat the oven to 180°C/350°F/Gas 4. Line 3 baking sheets with baking paper.

Combine all the dry ingredients in a large mixing bowl.

Put the vanilla extract, maple syrup and coconut oil in a saucepan and heat gently until the coconut oil melts and the mixture is runny. (This will help to distribute the mixture evenly through the dry ingredients.) Remove from the heat and pour the liquid over the dry ingredients. Stir thoroughly to combine.

Tip the granola on to the prepared baking sheets and spread out evenly. The baking sheets should only have a 2cm (¾in) thin layer of granola. Bake for 35 minutes, or until the granola is a deep golden brown.

Remove the granola from the oven and allow to cool completely on the baking sheets. The granola should be dry and not sticky. If sticky, bake the granola again at the same temperature for another 10 minutes, but be careful not to let it burn. The key to this granola keeping its characteristic clumps is to not touch or move the granola at any stage of its baking or cooling process.

Once cooled, break up the granola clumps with your fingers as needed. Store in an airtight container.

I am not a coffee drinker. My tipple of choice is a good cup of warm chai and, trust me, I don't let my obsession with this spice combination stop there. I love to incorporate it into my breakfasts and meals, too.

This porridge settles in your insides like a soft, warm blanket. It takes care of you and gives you a little pleasure when it's dark and frosty outside.

CHAI-SPICED PORRIDGE (v)

SERVES 2

100g (3½oz/1 cup) rolled oats
a pinch of sea salt
½ teaspoon ground cinnamon
¼ teaspoon ground nutmeg
a pinch of ground cardamom
¼ teaspoon ground ginger
440ml (15¼fl oz/scant 2 cups)
   oat milk, or milk of your choice
2 tablespoons pure maple syrup
2 tablespoons almond butter
1 teaspoon pure vanilla extract
full-fat, natural Greek yoghurt
   (vegan if necessary), to serve
Pick-me-up Cacao Granola
   (see page 143), to serve

Add the oats, salt and spices to a small saucepan and stir to combine, then add the milk and maple syrup. Place over a medium heat and gently bring to a steady simmer, then cook for 3–4 minutes, stirring occasionally.

Once the oats are tender and cooked, remove the pan from the heat and stir through the almond butter and vanilla extract. Stir to combine and divide between 2 breakfast bowls.

To serve, top with a dollop of yoghurt and a sprinkle of granola.

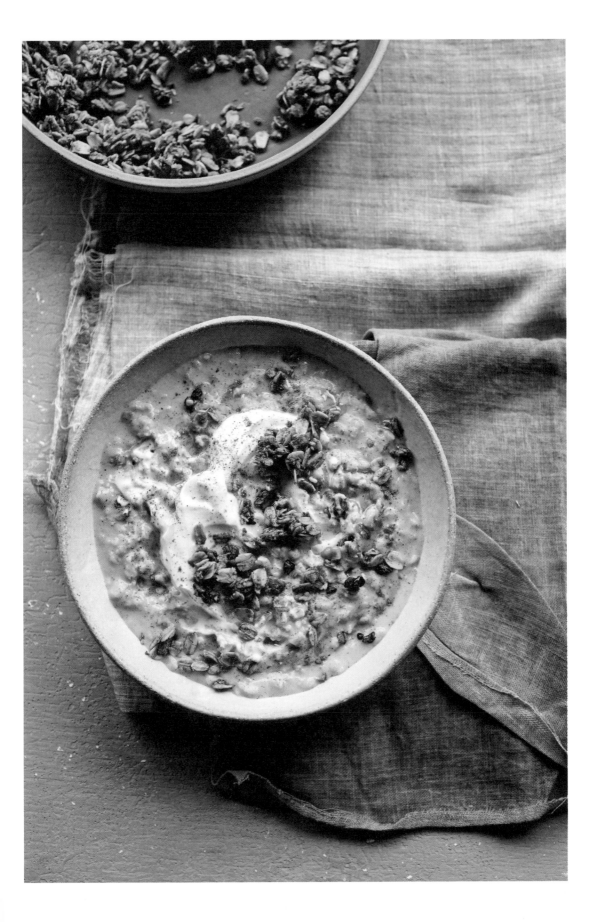

Cracked freekeh is harvested when the grain is still young and green, before the gluten-containing outer casing of the wheat grain forms, so it is a gluten-free form of wheat.

In this salad I have added the cracked freekeh to broccoli rice, along with traditional tabbouleh herbs to create a more interesting tabbouleh base.

Because the third-eye chakra is so connected to your brain's performance, I have offered omega-rich oils such as flaxseed, hemp and avocado as options other than olive oil to dress the tabbouleh. For a dose of predominantly omega-3s choose flaxseed; for a perfect ratio of omega 3,6 and 9 choose hemp; and for a dose of predominantly omega-9s choose avocado oil.

PISTACHIO & FREEKEH TABBOULEH
with blackberries & grilled halloumi crumbs

SERVES 2

FOR THE PISTACHIO &
FREEKEH TABBOULEH
80g (2¾oz/⅓ cup) cracked
    freekeh
½ head broccoli, chopped
    into florets
2 tablespoons apple cider vinegar
1 teaspoon honey
2 tablespoons extra virgin olive oil
30g (1oz/scant ¼ cup) raw
    pistachios, roughly chopped
3 mint sprigs, leaves picked and
    finely chopped
6 flat-leaf parsley sprigs, leaves
    picked and finely chopped
80g (2¾oz/1 cup) sugar snap
    peas, blanched and halved
200g (7oz) halloumi cheese
sea salt and cracked black pepper

TO SERVE
100g (3½oz/¾ cup) fresh
    blackberries, half chopped
    in half
flaxseed, hemp, avocado or olive
    oil, to drizzle (optional)

Put the freekeh in a medium saucepan with 250ml (9fl oz/1 cup) water and place over a high heat. Bring to the boil, cover with a lid and reduce the heat to low. Simmer for 10 minutes or until tender. Remove from the heat and place a clean tea towel over the saucepan, then, using the saucepan lid, try to create a seal so no steam is able to escape. Set aside to cool.

Meanwhile, place the broccoli florets in a food processor and blend until you have small grains. Transfer to a large mixing bowl and set aside.

Put the apple cider vinegar, honey and olive oil in a small bowl. Season with salt and pepper and whisk to combine.

Add the pistachios, mint, parsley, sugar snap peas and dressing to the broccoli grains. Add the cooled freekeh and stir to combine. Taste for seasoning and adjust as desired.

Place a non-stick frying pan over high heat. Crumble the halloumi into the pan and gently cook until golden. This will only take a few minutes. Remove from the pan and set aside.

To assemble, divide the freekeh tabbouleh between 2 plates and scatter with blackberries and the grilled halloumi crumbs. Drizzle with some extra oil of choice, if desired, and enjoy.

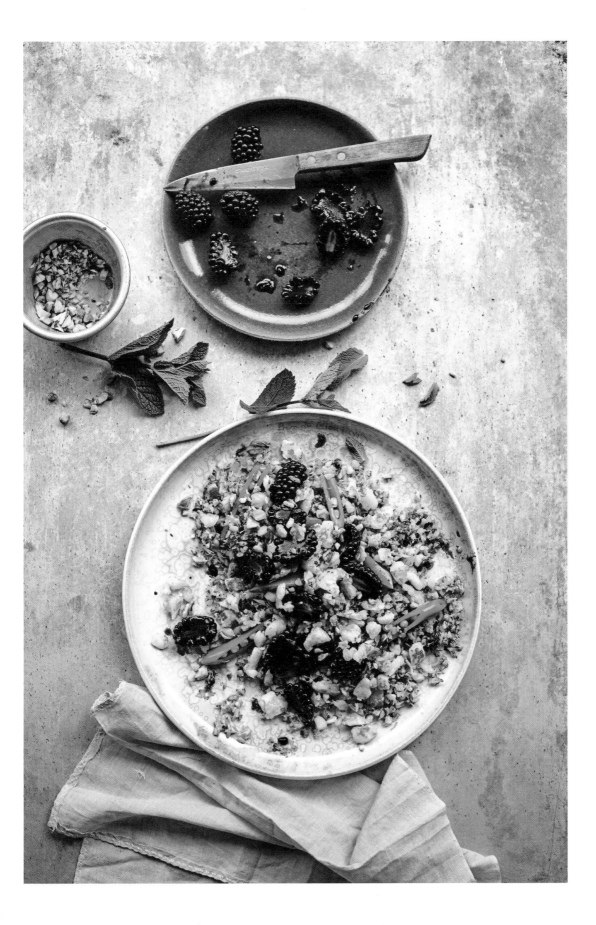

You'll be amazed how much this nut 'cheese' tastes just like a soft Cheddar. Although it may seem like a bit of work to make the cheese, I have really come to appreciate the art of making nut cheeses and I recommend giving it a go.

Serve for a dinner party starter or as a simple weekday lunch. This soup is suitable for simplicity or celebration.

NUT CHEESE WITH CHILLED BLACKBERRY SOUP (v)

SERVES 2

FOR THE NUT CHEESE

100g (3½oz/heaped ¾ cup) cashew nuts, soaked for at least 2 hours, drained and rinsed
½ teaspoon probiotic powder (you can use the powder from 2–3 probiotic capsules)
1 teaspoon white miso paste
3 tablespoons nutritional yeast flakes
1 teaspoon finely chopped chives
sea salt and cracked black pepper

FOR THE CHILLED BLACKBERRY SOUP

450g (1lb/3½ cups) fresh or frozen blackberries
½ large cucumber
1 tablespoon thyme leaves
2 tablespoons roughly chopped basil
2 teaspoons balsamic glaze
2 teaspoons maple syrup
60ml (2fl oz/¼ cup) extra virgin olive oil

TO SERVE

a few pinches of store-bought dukkah
crackers or crusty bread

Begin by making the nut cheese. Place the cashews, probiotic powder, miso paste and yeast flakes in a food processor and blitz until very smooth and creamy. Season with salt and pepper

Place a fine sieve over a large bowl and layer 2–3 pieces of kitchen towel into the sieve, or use a cheesecloth or muslin if you have one. Scoop the cheese mixture onto the kitchen towel or cheesecloth, then wrap it in a tight bundle and tie with a rubber band. Cover with cling film (plastic wrap) and let sit in the sieve at room temperature for 24–48 hours, so the cheese can ferment. After fermentation, place the cheese (still in the bundle) in the fridge for at least 2 hours, so it's easier to work with.

Preheat the oven to its lowest setting (approximately 50°C/120°F). Transfer the cheese to a bowl and stir in the chives. Spread the cheese into moulds of your choice, then turn out onto a baking sheet. Remove the moulds and place in the oven to dehydrate for 3–6 hours, or until dry to the touch.

Meanwhile make the blackberry soup. Combine the blackberries, cucumber, thyme, basil, balsamic glaze and maple syrup in a blender and blitz until smooth. Now blend for a further few minutes on a lower setting and drizzle in the olive oil. Season with salt and pepper, to taste. Pour through a sieve to remove the blackberry seeds, then chill for at least 1 hour, ideally longer.

To serve, place one cheese round into the middle of 2 shallow soup bowls. Pour the soup around the cheese and serve with a sprinkle of dukkah over . Serve with crackers or crusty bread.

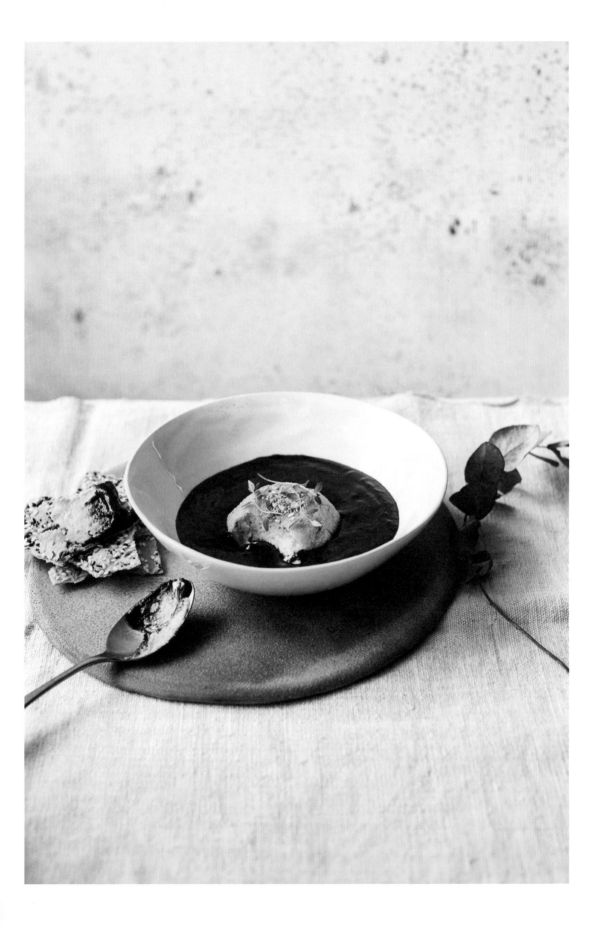

This started off as a roasted turmeric cauliflower recipe until I realized how much more vibrant the colour was when you boiled the cauliflower in turmeric-spiced water – it's fantastic and I still get a kick out of it every time I make it.

This was a salad we used to serve at my yoga cafés in London. Back then it came with a tahini dressing but over the years I have begun to enjoy it without the need for a dressing. I've simplified its components so that you really get to taste the sweet coconut and sultanas along with the cauliflower, chickpeas and carrot. But if you would like to add a dressing, go ahead and put together a simple tahini and honey-based dressing.

TURMERIC CAULIFLOWER, CARROT & CHICKPEA SALAD
with sweet coconut & sultanas (v)

SERVES 2

½ teaspoon ground turmeric
½ head cauliflower, florets removed and cut into bite-size pieces
2 carrots, peeled and grated
200g (7oz/1½ cups) canned chickpeas (garbanzo beans), rinsed and drained
20g (⅔oz/heaped ⅓ cup) desiccated (dried shredded) coconut
40g (1½oz/heaped ¼ cup) sultanas (golden raisins)
2 tablespoons roughly chopped coriander (cilantro) leaves
1 handful rocket (arugula) leaves
sea salt and cracked black pepper
black sesame seeds, to serve
toasted cashew nuts, to serve

Bring a saucepan of water to the boil, then add the turmeric and the cauliflower florets. Bring the liquid back to a rolling simmer and cook the cauliflower for 2–3 minutes. Remove from the heat and strain through a colander immediately. The cauliflower will be a vibrant yellow colour.

Put the carrots, chickpeas, coconut and sultanas in a mixing bowl. Add the turmeric cauliflower and toss to combine. Season to taste with salt and black pepper. Now add the coriander and rocket leaves and carefully fold all the ingredients together.

Serve the salad with a scattering of black sesame seeds and toasted cashew nuts.

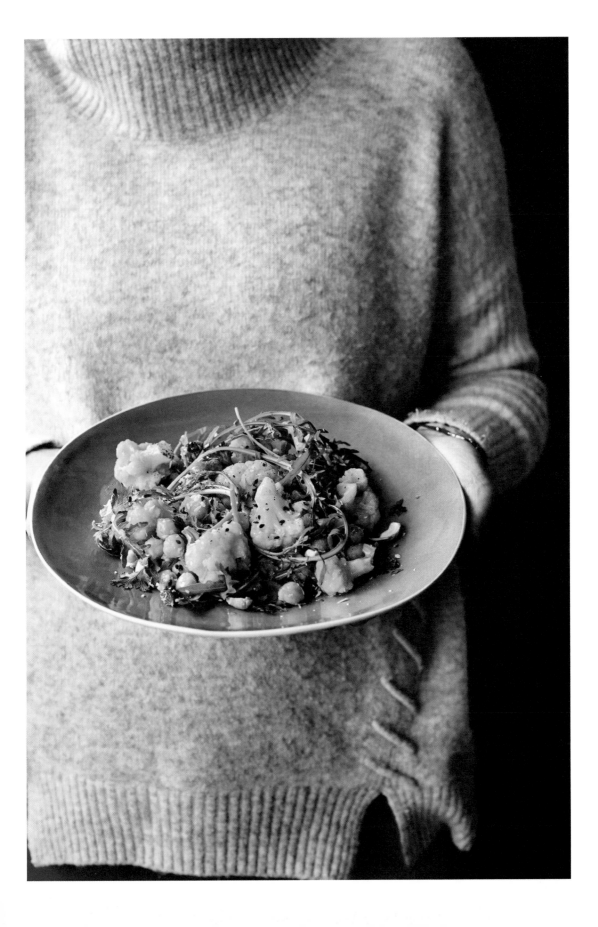

Ricotta on toast has been a regular breakfast staple my whole life. I usually enjoy it whipped with some honey and dolloped on a piece of thick, crusty toast. I wanted to pay homage to it, change it up a little and create a lunchtime snack that brings simple ingredients together in a sophisticated way.

I am happy to say I think I achieved it with these bruschette. They are elegant while also simple to prepare and that's always what I strive for in my cooking.

RICOTTA, ROASTED GRAPES & THYME BRUSCHETTA

SERVES 2

250g (9oz) red grapes
extra virgin olive oil, for drizzling
   and brushing
sea salt, for sprinkling
4 thyme sprigs
4 slices sourdough bread
200g (7oz/scant 1 cup) ricotta
   cheese
2 tablespoons flaked (slivered)
   almonds

Preheat the oven to 200°C/400°F/Gas 6.

Spread the grapes out on a baking sheet. Drizzle with olive oil and sprinkle with sea salt. Lay the thyme sprigs over the top of the grapes. Toss everything together gently with your hands. Bake in the preheated oven for 7 minutes, or until the grapes' skins are just about to break and crack.

Meanwhile, heat a grill (broiler) to medium–high or a griddle (char-grill) pan over medium–high heat. Brush the bread with olive oil. Grill (broil) or griddle until nice and toasted.

Assemble the sourdough toasts by spreading fresh ricotta over each piece of bread, then top with roasted grapes and toasted almonds and serve.

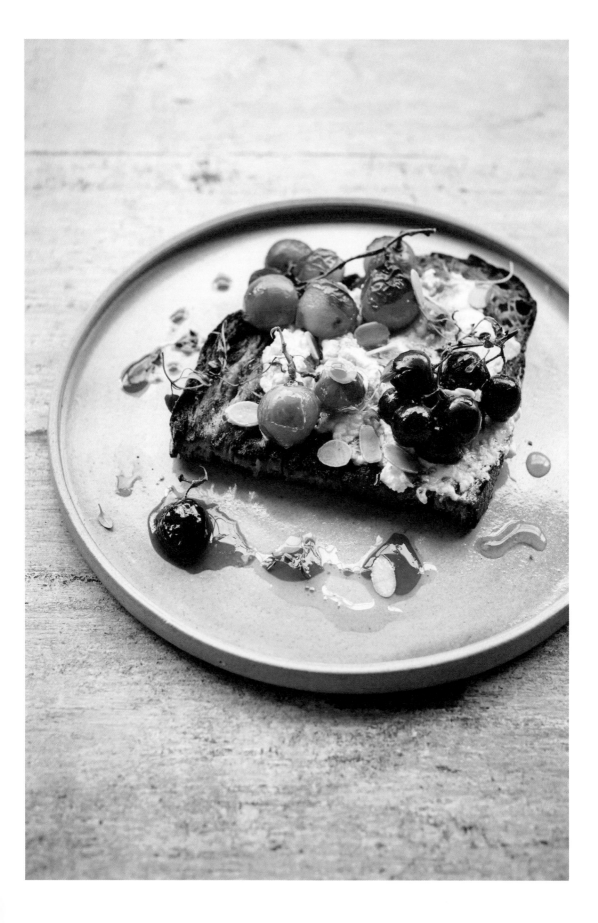

The aromas in your kitchen as you start to prepare the spices in this dish will transport you to the streets of the East. If there were ever a recipe that seemed more yogic than others, it would have to be a wholesome bowl of dhal. Simple in its appearance and texture, but big on flavour.

This is a great recipe to double or triple in quantity to store some wholesome meals away in the freezer bank. I never tire of this dhal, and I think it has something to do with the curry leaves and mustard seed combination. They are spices I rarely use except in this dish. I just keep coming back for more and more of this dhal and I hope you will, too.

ROASTED TOMATO & SPINACH DHAL (v)

SERVES 2

220g (7¾oz) plum, vine tomatoes, washed and halved
1 tablespoon extra virgin olive oil
1 teaspoon cumin seeds
1½ teaspoons black mustard seeds
5–6 curry leaves
2 celery sticks, finely diced
200g (7oz/heaped 1 cup) split red lentils, washed and drained several times
1 teaspoon ground turmeric
½ teaspoon sea salt
5 tablespoons full-fat coconut milk
70g (2½oz/1 heaped cup) spinach
full-fat, natural Greek yoghurt (vegan if necessary), to serve
toasted flaked (slivered) almonds, to serve

Preheat the oven to 200°C/400°F/Gas 6.

Place the tomatoes in a roasting tray in which they can lie in a single layer. Sprinkle with a pinch of salt and roast for 45 minutes, or until slightly shrunken and charred in places.

Heat the olive oil in a medium, heavy-based saucepan, add the cumin, mustard seeds and curry leaves and allow to sizzle over a medium–high heat. You should hear the mustard and cumin seeds start to pop. The spices will be very aromatic and your kitchen will be filled with the lovely aromas too. After 4–5 minutes, add the celery and lower the heat to medium. Gently sauté the celery for 4–5 minutes, then add the lentils, turmeric and 450ml (16fl oz/2 cups) water. Stir to combine, cover the saucepan with a lid and cook for 15–20 minutes or until the lentils are cooked through. Now add the ½ teaspoon sea salt and the coconut milk and stir to combine again. Taste for seasoning and adjust if necessary.

Remove the dhal from the heat, add the spinach and roasted tomatoes and stir them through.

Divide the dhal between 2 serving bowls. Top each bowl with a dollop of yoghurt and the toasted almonds. Enjoy while piping hot.

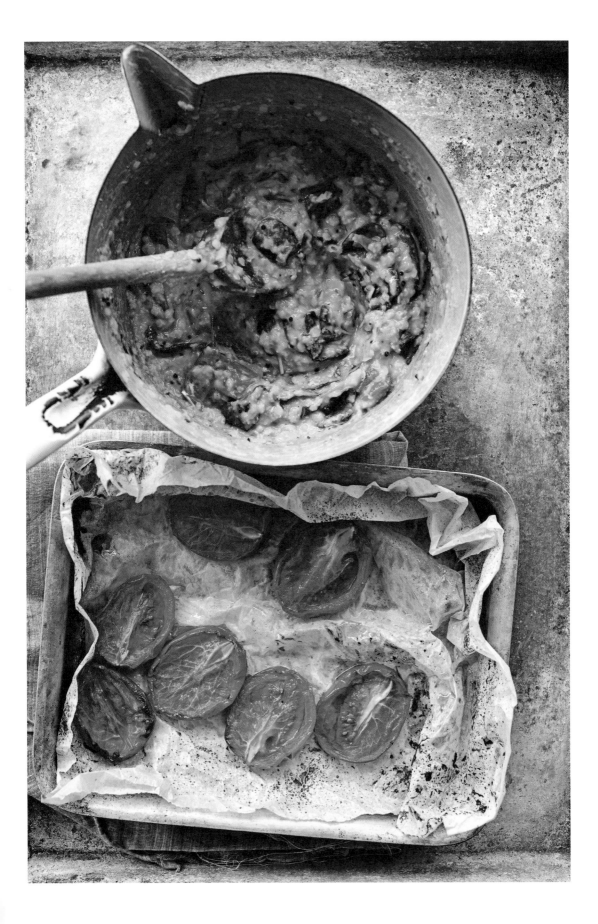

For when that pasta craving hits! This clever vegetable upgrade banishes the empty carbs of pasta and fills your plate with lush vegetables while still retaining all the aromatic flavours of a traditional pasta dish.

COURGETTI PUTTANESCA (v)

SERVES 2

300g (10oz) baby heirloom
   tomatoes
1 long red chilli, halved
1 lemon, halved
2 tablespoons extra virgin olive oil
½ teaspoon sea salt flakes
200g (7oz/2 cups) drained
   canned artichokes
600g (1lb 5oz) courgettes
   (zucchini), spiralized or thinly
   sliced lengthways using a
   julienne peeler
130g (4¾oz/1¼ cups) mixed
   pitted olives
1 tablespoon nutritional yeast
   flakes
6 flat-leaf parsley sprigs, leaves
   picked and roughly chopped
cracked black pepper

Preheat the oven to 180°C/350°F/Gas 4.

Place the tomatoes, chilli and lemon on a large baking sheet and drizzle with the olive oil. Season with the salt and pepper, then cook for 15–20 minutes or until the tomatoes are blistered and soft.

Add the artichokes, courgettes and olives to the sheet, toss to combine and return to the oven for 3 minutes to warm through.

Sprinkle over the nutritional yeast and parsley and toss to combine, then serve.

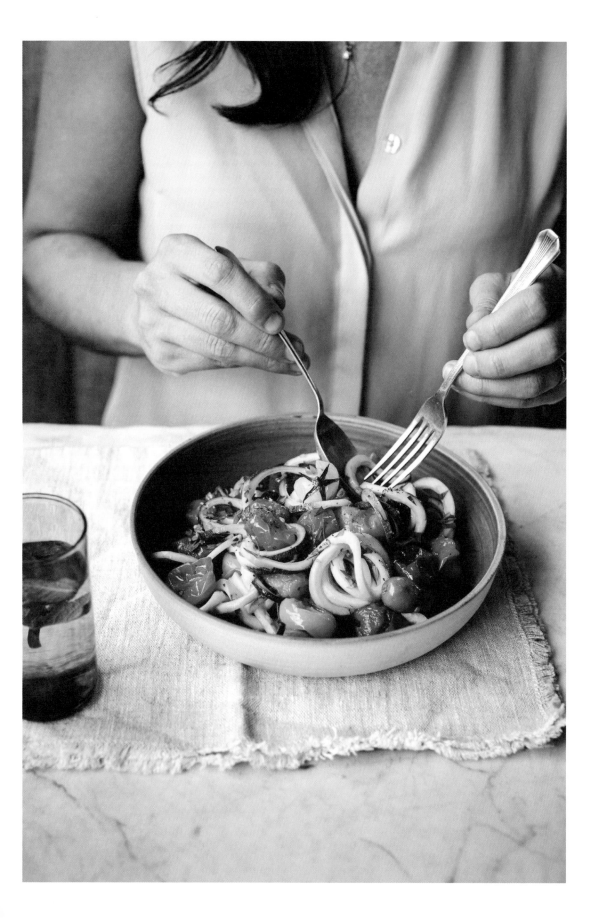

It is truly amazing what you can do with a couple of cans of beans. Their versatility was unveiled to me when I visited a friend who had just returned from a trip to Sardinia; she told me about a meal she had enjoyed in a simple taverna on the beach one summer's evening. She wanted to recreate it in her kitchen back in London with me, so we did and I have to thank her for this magic recipe.

Flageolet beans are a member of the haricot bean family; they are picked before the beans are ripe and retain their green colour and they are even more flavourful than a regular cannellini or haricot bean. You can buy them pre-cooked in cans in most supermarkets or you can substitute with butter beans or any other white bean you like.

RADICCHIO, GRAPE & BALSAMIC TRAY BAKE
with bean & rosemary purée (v)

SERVES 2

1 head of radicchio
1 fennel bulb, finely sliced
2 bunches red grapes, about 200g (7oz) in total
2½ tablespoons extra virgin olive oil
2½ tablespoons balsamic vinegar
1 teaspoon dried thyme (or leaves from 3 thyme sprigs)
sea salt and cracked black pepper

FOR THE BEAN PURÉE

1 sprig rosemary
2 x 400g (14oz) cans flageolet beans, drained and rinsed
½ vegetable stock cube
1 tablespoon extra virgin olive oil

Preheat the oven to 180°C/350°F/Gas 4.

Halve the head of radicchio, then cut each half into four sections. Trim the base and a little of the white heart from each piece, without letting the sections fall apart. Place onto a baking sheet. Scatter the fennel slices over the top of the radicchio, then add the grape bunches to the baking sheet. Pour over the olive oil and balsamic vinegar, then scatter the thyme leaves over as well. Season with salt and pepper. Bake in the preheated oven for 30 minutes until the grape skins have split and the radicchio and fennel are soft.

In the meantime, prepare the bean purée by placing all the ingredients into a blender or food processor with 150ml (5fl oz/scant ⅔ cup) boiling water and blending on high speed until smooth. Taste for seasoning.

To serve, place a dollop of the bean purée in the centre of each plate, then spoon the baked vegetables over the top. Drizzle the balsamic juices from the baking sheet over the top of each plate and enjoy immediately.

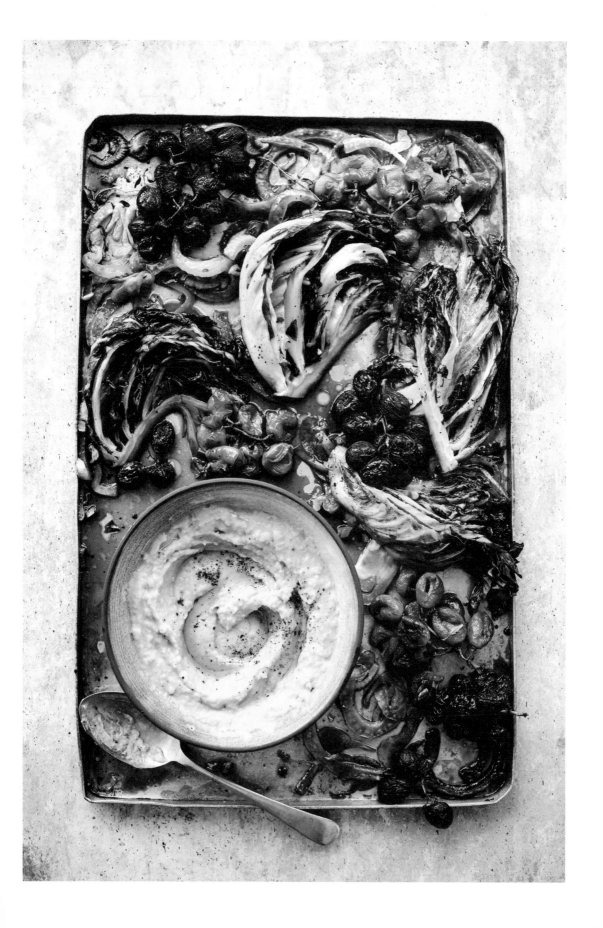

As the gatekeeper of your spiritual potential, the third-eye chakra is connected to your ability to trust your intuition, and to join your mental, emotional, spiritual and physical bodies to each other and to this world.

An out-of-balance third-eye chakra can lead to a foggy, tired and indecisive state of mind. You may feel disoriented and disconnected from everything going on around you and describe yourself as feeling 'numb'. Your tendencies may be to procrastinate, forget, struggle to concentrate, and feel fearful more often than not. On the other hand, if you have too much energy here, it's likely that your mind is constantly in overdrive.

TERIYAKI CAULIFLOWER BITES
with brown rice & grilled pineapple red cabbage cups (v)

SERVES 2

FOR THE BROWN
RICE CUPS

¼ large pineapple, trimmed
   and peeled
olive oil, for brushing
500g brown rice, cooked
1 tablespoon toasted sesame oil
1 tablespoon mirin
2 tablespoons tamari sauce
140g (5oz/1 cup) frozen
   edamame beans, thawed
1 sheet nori seaweed cut in half
   and then half again, then into
   thin strips

FOR THE
CAULIFLOWER BITES

1 head of cauliflower
2 tablespoons sweet chilli sauce
3 tablespoons teriyaki sauce
1 tablespoon mirin
2 tablespoons coconut sugar

TO SERVE

4 whole red cabbage leaves
   or lettuce leaves
70g (2½oz/scant ½ cup) pickled
   ginger slices

Heat a ridged griddle (char-grill) pan over a very high heat. Cut the trimmed pineapple into 4 thin slices – about 5mm (¼in) thick – then brush them with a thin layer of olive oil on each side. Place into the hot pan and cook for 2 minutes on each side. The pineapple should take on the characteristic charred grill lines when it's ready. If you don't get the grill lines, then your grill isn't hot enough and you need to increase the temperature. Remove the pineapple from the pan and place to one side.

To prepare the cauliflower, place a saucepan of water over a high heat and bring to the boil. Cut the cauliflower into florets and, once boiling, add the florets to the saucepan. Bring the water back to the boil, then strain immediately through a colander.

Place the sweet chilli and teriyaki sauces, the mirin and coconut sugar into a large non-stick frying pan over a medium heat. Stir to combine and dissolve coconut sugar, allow to simmer gently for 1 minute, then add the cauliflower florets to the pan. Coat the cauliflower in the sauce and cook for 5 minutes stirring regularly to make sure the cauliflower doesn't overcook. Remove from the heat and set aside while you prepare the brown rice.

In a mixing bowl, add the cooked rice and the remaining rice-cup ingredients and stir to combine.

To serve, take a red cabbage leaf and place a slice of grilled pineapple to one side inside the leaf. Add 3 tablespoons brown rice, a few cauliflower florets and some pickled ginger slices. Repeat for the 3 other red cabbage leaves and serve.

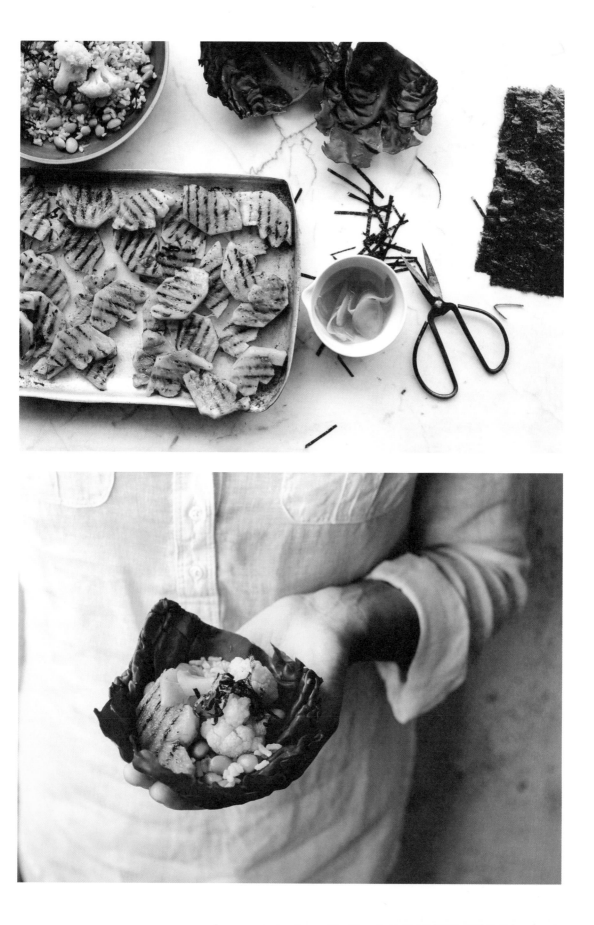

CROWN CHAKRA

connection

Key foods for the crown chakra:
WHITE FOOD: fennel, pear, cauliflower, coconut
LIGHT, VERY EASY-TO-DIGEST FOOD:
sprouts, grapefruit, lemon, pomelo
MOSTLY LIQUIDS: tea, juice, smoothie
DETOXIFYING FOOD: aloe vera
Enjoy small portions and avoid dense, heavy food

There is something about these smoothies that quietens my mind whenever I make them, which is why these recipes are so perfectly placed here for the crown chakra. Finding the peace that already exists in your mind is often an initial hurdle you have to overcome when seeking to reach a state of meditation or connecting to your higher conscious. These smoothies help you get there with blissful ease.

When making the first smoothie, if pears aren't in season, you can use canned pears and if you want less sweetness you can substitute the apple juice for water or grapefruit, which I sometimes do for something a little more tart.

BIRD OF PARADISE PEAR, GINGER & COCONUT MILK SMOOTHIE (v)

SERVES 2

2 ripe pears, cored
1 banana, peeled
2 thick slices of peeled ginger
4 tablespoons coconut milk
450ml (16fl oz/scant 2 cups) fresh apple juice
freshly squeezed juice of 1 lime

Blitz all the ingredients together in a blender for 2–3 minutes.

Pour into 2 glasses and enjoy.

SUMMER LOVE SMOOTHIE (v)

SERVES 2

1 fresh or frozen avocado, peeled and pitted
4 slices of fresh pineapple, peeled and cored
1 lime, peeled
8 mint leaves
6 lychees, peeled and deseeded
1 tablespoon flaxseed oil
450ml (16fl oz/scant 2 cups) coconut water

Blitz all the ingredients together in a blender for 2–3 minutes.

Pour into 2 glasses and enjoy.

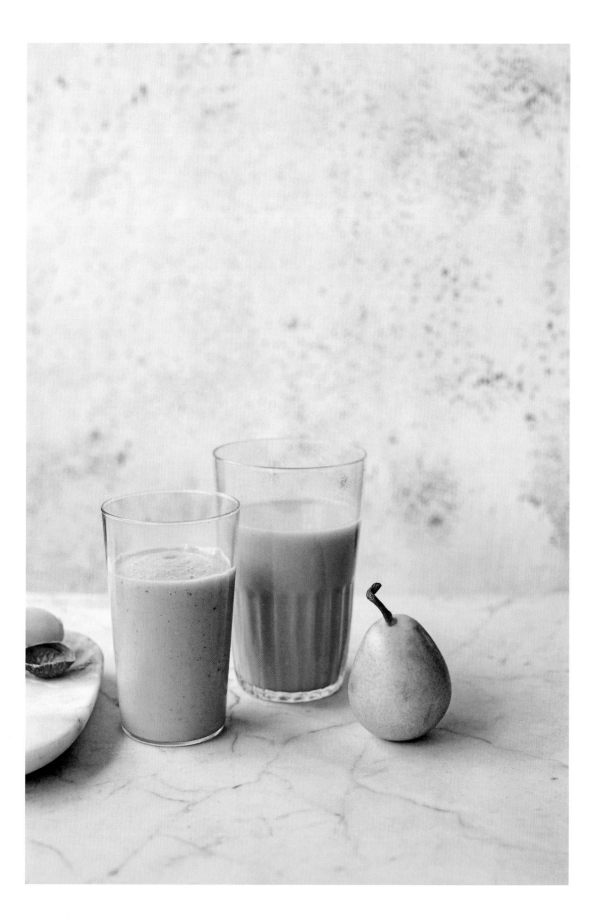

Somewhere between a Waldorf and a Caesar salad, this is a great example of how I like to cook. I am terrible at following a recipe to the letter, preferring to manipulate recipes so that they take on a new twist.

Here I have taken the two ingredients I love from a Waldorf salad – apple and walnuts – and twisted them into a Caesar salad, which has new life with a creamy, vegan pine-nut dressing and crispy chickpeas in place of traditional croutons.

YOGI CAESAR SALAD
with pine-nut dressing & crispy chickpea croutons (v)

SERVES 2

FOR THE DRESSING

50g (1¾oz/heaped ⅓ cup) pine nuts/kernels, soaked in filtered water for 2 hours
2 tablespoons apple cider vinegar
2½ tablespoons extra virgin olive oil
½ teaspoon sea salt
½ teaspoon ground sumac, plus extra to garnish
1 tablespoon nutritional yeast flakes
2 tablespoons filtered water

FOR THE CRISPY CHICKPEA CROUTONS

2 teaspoons extra virgin olive oil
1 x 400g (14oz) can chickpeas (garbanzo beans), rinsed and drained
1 teaspoon sweet paprika
1 teaspoon ground sumac
pinch of sea salt

FOR THE SALAD

½ cos lettuce or 1 small baby gem (Bibb) lettuce
¼ cucumber, cut into thin rounds
½ Granny Smith apple, cored and julienned
4 radishes, thinly sliced into rounds
½ avocado, pitted, peeled and thinly sliced
2 tablespoons roasted walnuts

First make the dressing. Drain the pine nuts and place them in a blender or food processor. Add the vinegar, olive oil, salt, sumac and yeast flakes, and, with the motor running, pour the water through the feed tube, a splash at a time, to achieve the desired consistency. Set aside.

For the crispy chickpea croutons, heat the olive oil in a large frying pan over a high heat. Add the chickpeas, sweet paprika, sumac and sea salt and cook, stirring, for 8 minutes or until the chickpeas are crisp. Remove from the heat and set aside.

To prepare the salad, wash 6 lettuce leaves and pat dry with some kitchen towel. Divide between 2 serving plates, overlapping the lettuce leaves in the middle of each plate. Then scatter the cucumber, julienned apple, radishes and crispy chickpeas over the lettuce leaves. Drizzle a few tablespoons of the dressing over the salad, then place a few slices of avocado on top. Scatter a few walnuts around the plate and serve.

The dressing will keep in the fridge for 2–3 days or can be frozen for the next time you want to make this salad.

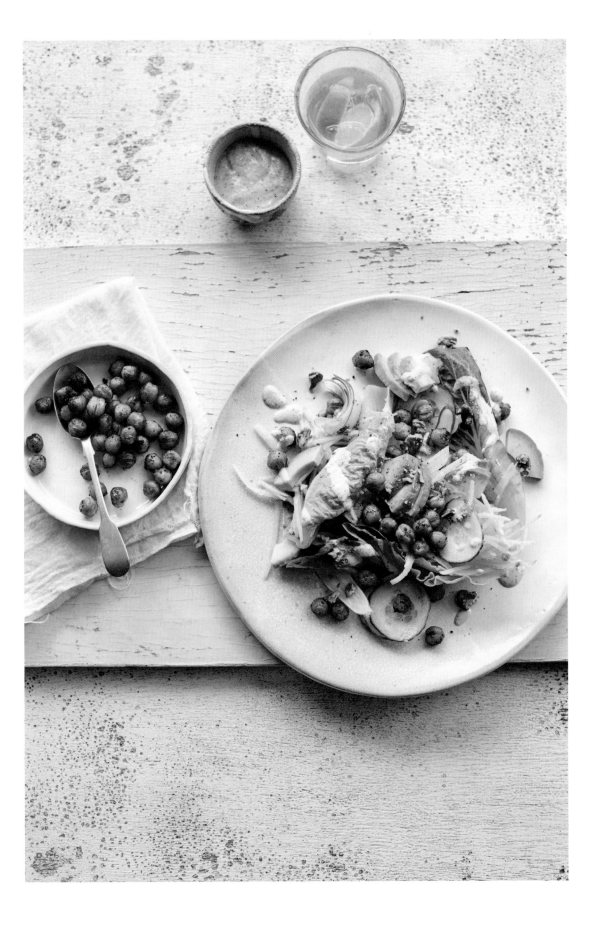

Don't you just love how soup chases away chills, soothes the soul, nurtures the appetite and leaves you feeling warm and loved all over? I do!

This soup won't blow you away with robust flavours; it's far more subtle than that and I think that is its overall charm.

BROCCOLI, CORIANDER & WHITE MISO SOUP (v)

SERVES 2

500g (1lb 2 oz) frozen broccoli florets, or 1 head of fresh broccoli, chopped into florets
250g (9oz/2 cups) frozen peas
500ml (17fl oz/2 cups) vegetable stock
leaves from 5 coriander (cilantro) sprigs
200ml (7fl oz/generous ¾ cup) canned full-fat coconut milk
2 tablespoons coconut butter
2 teaspoons white miso paste
hulled hemp seeds, to serve
coconut milk, to drizzle

Put the broccoli florets, peas and vegetable stock into a large saucepan. Place over a high heat and bring to the boil. Reduce the heat to a gentle simmer. Cover and cook for approximately 3–5 minutes or until the broccoli is cooked but still al dente.

Remove from the heat and let sit for 5 minutes to cool slightly. Add the coriander leaves, coconut milk, coconut butter and miso paste. Transfer to a blender or use a stick blender to purée the soup until smooth.

Serve the soup with a sprinkle of hemp seeds and a drizzle of coconut milk.

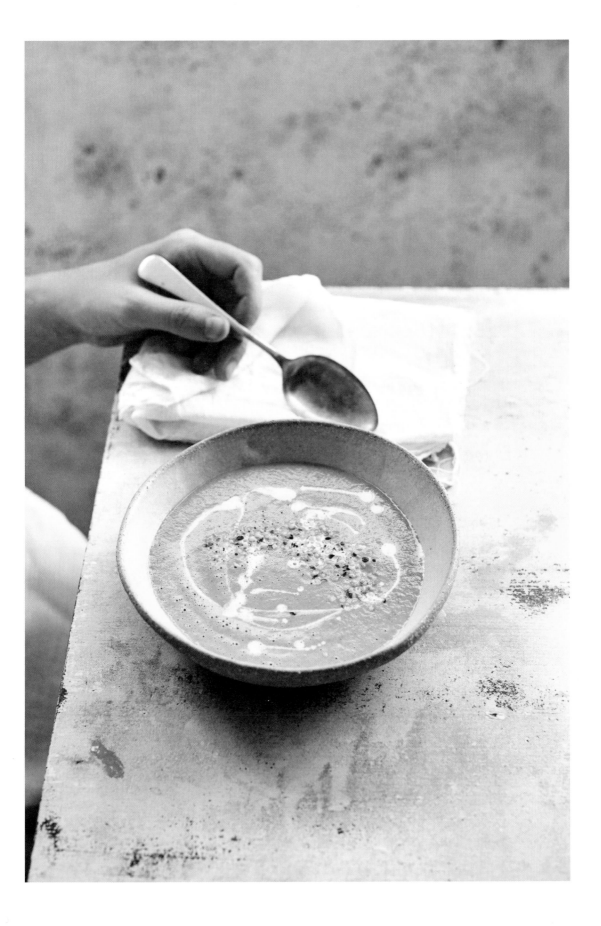

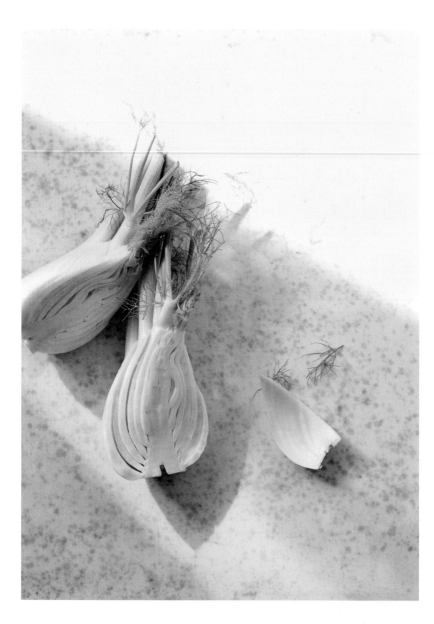

I SEE BEYOND MY LIMITING BELIEFS AND ACCEPT
MY HUMAN EXPERIENCE FULLY.

I HONOUR MY BODY AS THE TEMPLE THAT
NOURISHES MY SOUL.

Highly spiritual, the crown chakra is about self-realization and the connection with the world around us. It focuses on seeking wisdom and understanding, so when choosing foods for this chakra you should focus more on fasting and detoxing rather than the kinds of foods used to build and maintain our body's strength and stamina.

This broth has a great flavour and I love making large quantities to freeze for the rainy days when a warm mug of aromatic broth is exactly what I feel like. Healing to your gut, ginger is the surprise hero that makes this such a special mug of goodness. Meanwhile the other ingredients, such as fennel, seaweed and mushrooms, are so subtle but highly important for the synergy of this broth to work.

BONELESS GUT-HEALING BROTH (v)

SERVES 2

1 tablespoon coconut oil
a 2.5cm (1in) piece of ginger, peeled and roughly sliced
1 small fennel bulb, plus fronds, roughly chopped
1 large carrot, roughly chopped
1 celery stick, roughly chopped
½ leek, roughly chopped
150g (5½oz) whole chestnut (cremini) mushrooms
50g (1¾oz/2 cups) dried shiitake mushrooms
15g (½oz) dried wakame seaweed (or other seaweed variety)
3 black peppercorns
¼ teaspoon ground turmeric
1 tablespoon tamari sauce
2 flat-leaf parsley sprigs
2 coriander (cilantro) sprigs
1 tablespoon nutritional yeast flakes
750ml (26fl oz/3 cups) filtered water
freshly squeezed juice of ½ lime
sea salt

Place all the ingredients, except the lime juice and salt, into a large heavy-based saucepan. Slowly bring the contents to the boil over a low–medium heat. Once simmering, cover with a lid and allow to simmer over a low heat for 1 hour.

Once the broth has simmered for 1 hour, remove from the heat and strain through a fine sieve or muslin cloth. Add the lime juice and season to taste.

Serve in a large mug and enjoy the warming aromas immediately.

If you prefer, you can cool the broth completely and store it in an airtight container in the fridge for up to 5 days or freeze for those moments when a hot mug of broth is just what you need.

I know, another courgetti recipe! I refrained from featuring this recipe in the original *The Yoga Kitchen* book because I didn't want to be one of *those* healthy chefs. But I have been serving this recipe on my yoga retreats for the last 3 years and it's always such a crowd pleaser, so I just had to include it this time!

The sauce is creamy, light and slightly spicy, so for a milder sauce you can omit the dried chilli. The ginger is worth keeping though. It's a great dish if you want to recreate your very own *Lady and the Tramp* moment!

ZEN MANGO, AVOCADO COURGETTI BOWL (v)

SERVES 2

2 courgettes (zucchini)
thinly sliced radishes, to serve

FOR THE MANGO & AVOCADO SAUCE

1 medium fresh mango, peeled
   and trimmed from the stone,
   1 cup frozen mango pieces or
   ½ a 400g (14oz) can mango
   slices in juice, drained
1 avocado, peeled and pitted
leaves from 5 mint sprigs
½ teaspoon dried chilli
   (hot pepper) flakes
a 2.5cm (1in) piece of ginger,
   peeled
2 tablespoons tamari sauce
6 tablespoons canned full-fat
   coconut milk
sea salt and cracked black pepper

Wash the courgettes and spiralize them into a large mixing bowl. Set aside.

Place all the ingredients for the mango and avocado sauce into a blender and blend until smooth and creamy. Season to taste with salt and pepper.

Pour the sauce over the courgetti and toss to coat the courgetti using your hands.

To serve, arrange half of the courgetti on each plate and garnish with a few radish slices on top of each. Enjoy.

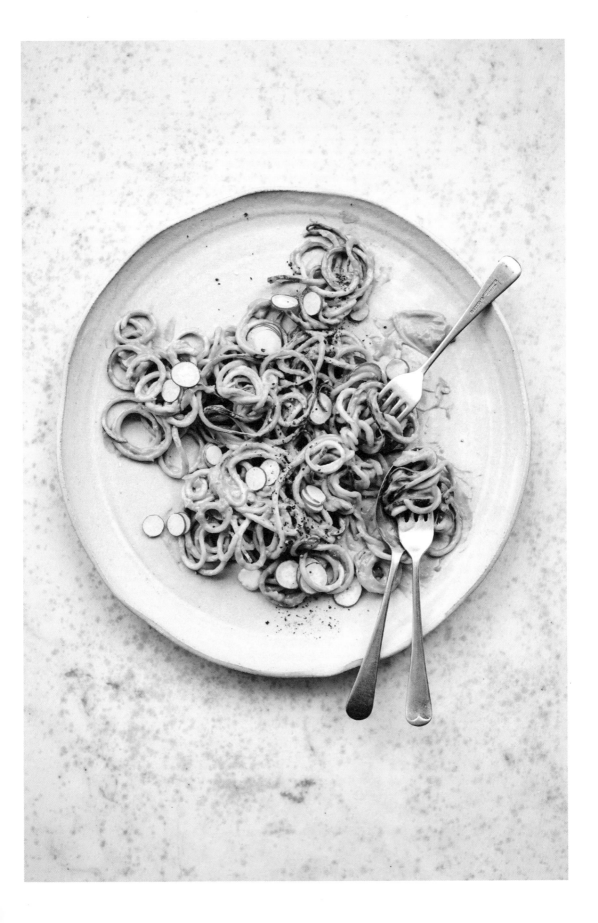

Eating is not just about sating appetite, but about appreciating with all your senses what is put before you, and honouring the ingredients with which it is made.

In this sushi recipe, we honour the plant kingdom and replace traditional sushi rice with a mix of broccoli, avocado and podded peas to create a sticky texture to encase the rest of the sushi ingredients.

Best eaten immediately, the sushi won't keep for long, so make sure you prepare them just prior to your meal.

BRO-SUSHI (v)

SERVES 2

3 tablespoons teriyaki sauce
3 portobello mushrooms (about (150g/5½oz), stalks removed
4 nori sheets
50g (1¾oz/scant 1 cup) spinach leaves, washed
¼ courgette (zucchini), julienned
½ carrot, peeled and julienned
½ teaspoon sesame seeds
tamari sauce

FOR THE BROCCOLI RICE

1 large head of broccoli, stem included
100g (3½oz/⅔ cup) frozen garden peas, thawed
flesh of 1 large avocado
20g (⅔oz/1 cup) coriander (cilantro), roughly chopped
2 mint sprigs, leaves picked
freshly squeezed juice and grated zest of ½ lime

To make the broccoli rice, remove the broccoli florets from the stem, then trim and peel the stem and roughly chop. Wash the broccoli, then add it to a food processor and pulse until a rice-like texture is reached. Add the peas, avocado, herbs and lime juice and zest and pulse again until combined. Remove the broccoli rice mixture from the food processor and set aside.

Place a frying pan over a low heat and add the teriyaki sauce and the Portobello mushrooms, open face down in the pan. Cover with a lid and allow the mushrooms to soften in the teriyaki sauce and lightly steam. Remove the pan from the heat and chop the mushrooms into thick slices.

To make the sushi, place a nori sheet on a sushi mat or flexible cutting board if you don't have a sushi mat. Starting from the bottom of the nori sheet, add a quarter of the broccoli mixture and spread it out to cover three-quarters of the nori sheet, leaving a bare strip at the top. Gently flatten the broccoli mixture to make sure it is evenly distributed and the mixture goes all the way to the edges of the nori sheet.

Place a layer of spinach leaves over the bottom quarter of the nori sheet and then add the Portobello mushrooms, courgette and carrot in a strip along the bottom edge of the nori sheet.

Now, gently but tightly, start to roll the sushi from the bottom of the sheet upwards, sealing the bare end of the nori sheet with a little dab of water. Repeat 3 more times, using the remaining nori sheets and ingredients.

In a small dipping bowl, stir the sesame seeds into the tamari.

To serve, cut the rolls into even bite-size pieces or in half for longer hand rolls. Dip into tamari and enjoy while fresh.

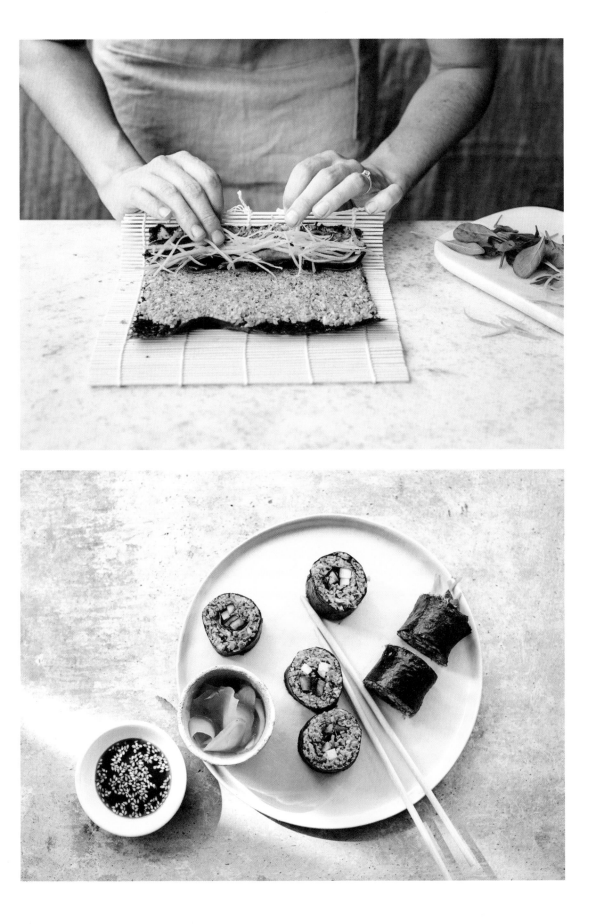

My first experience of shakshouka was on a trip to Israel where I devoured a rich tomato-based skillet of beans and spinach. While I dunked crusty bread into the thick sauce, I found myself considering all the different bean and flavour combinations that shakshouka could be adapted to. Moving away from the traditional tomato base, I found myself drawn to the idea of using white beans and pairing them with a creamy sauce and floral herbs, such as tarragon. Topped with the zest of lemon and the crunch of walnuts, this is my way of making a hot skillet of creamy beans and vegetables into the ultimate comfort food.

Replace the avocado with fried tofu for a completely hot dish.

CREAMY TARRAGON, PEA & SPINACH SHAKSHOUKA
with gremolata

SERVES 2

1 tablespoon extra virgin olive oil, plus extra to drizzle
1 celery stick, finely diced
1 teaspoon fennel seeds
3 tablespoons crème fraîche, or oat or soya cream
1 x 400g (14oz) can cannellini beans or white haricot beans, drained and rinsed
100g (3½oz/¾ cup) fresh or frozen peas (thawed if using frozen)
freshly squeezed juice of 1 lemon
100g (3½oz/2 cups) baby spinach leaves
1 tablespoon roughly chopped tarragon
sea salt and cracked black pepper
1 avocado, halved, pitted and peeled, to serve

FOR THE GREMOLATA

1 tablespoon finely chopped flat-leaf parsley
1 tablespoon finely chopped raw walnuts
freshly grated zest of ½ lemon

Heat the olive oil in a large cast iron skillet or heavy-based pan over a medium heat. Add the diced celery and fennel seeds and cook, stirring frequently, until the celery has softened, about 4–5 minutes.

Add the crème fraîche or cream of your choice, beans and peas to the pan, cover with a lid and bring to a light simmer. Reduce the heat to low and add the lemon juice and spinach to the pan, cover again and allow the spinach to wilt slightly. Remove from the heat and stir through the tarragon. Season with sea salt and black pepper to your taste.

To make the gremolata, place the parsley, walnuts and lemon zest into a small bowl and mix together.

To serve, spoon the shakshuka onto 2 plates, top with an avocado half and then sprinkle each serving with the gremolata. Let the zesty aromas hit your senses. Drizzle with a little extra virgin olive oil and serve immediately.

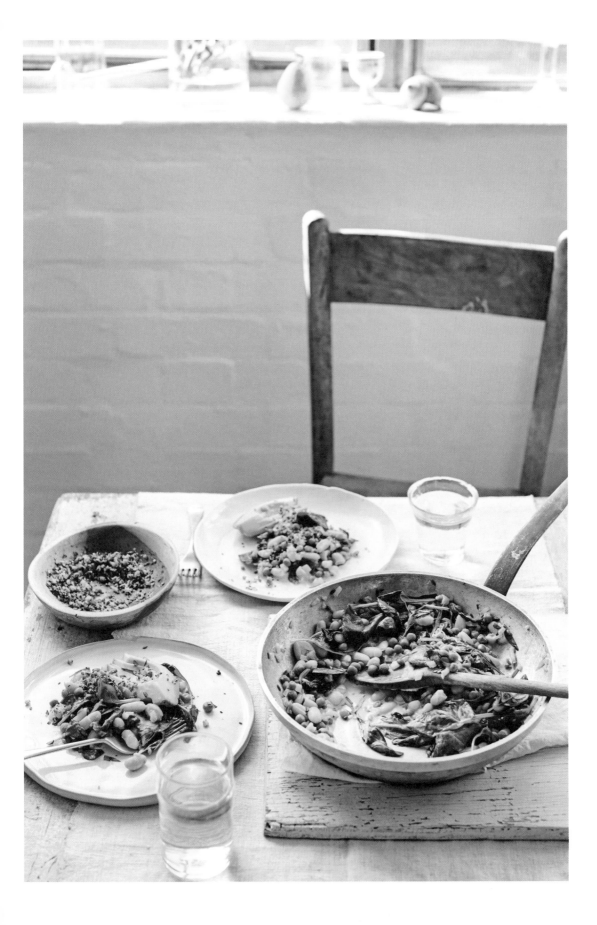

DAILY ELIXIRS

BEETROOT & GINGER

SERVES 1

¼ raw beetroot (beet), roughly chopped
1cm (½in) piece of ginger, peeled
100ml (3½fl oz/scant ½ cup) pomegranate, cranberry or orange juice, or water

Place all the ingredients in a high-speed blender or NutriBullet and blend for at least 1 minute. Sieve the elixir through a fine sieve over a jug, then serve in a small glass.

PINK GRAPEFRUIT, LEMON & GINGER

SERVES 1

½ lemon, peeled and deseeded
1cm (½in) piece of ginger, peeled
100ml (3½fl oz/scant ½ cup) pink grapefruit juice, or ½ fresh grapefruit, peeled, and 100ml (3½fl oz/scant ½ cup) water

Place all the ingredients in a high-speed blender or NutriBullet and blend for at least 1 minute. Sieve the elixir through a fine sieve over a jug, then serve in a small glass.

LEMON, PINEAPPLE, TURMERIC & BLACK PEPPER

SERVES 1

½ lemon, peeled and deseeded
1cm (½in) piece of fresh turmeric, peeled, or ½ teaspoon ground turmeric
1cm (½in) slice of pineapple, peeled, cored and roughly chopped
2 twists of cracked black pepper

Place all the ingredients in a high-speed blender or NutriBullet with 5 tablespoons water and blend for at least 1 minute. Sieve the elixir through a fine sieve over a jug, then serve in a small glass.

APPLE & WHEATGRASS

SERVES 1

100ml (3½fl oz/scant ½ cup)
   cloudy apple juice
½ teaspoon wheatgrass powder

Place all ingredients in a high-speed blender or NutriBullet and blend for at least 1 minute. Sieve the elixir through a fine sieve over a jug, then serve in a small glass.

SPIRULINA & STRAWBERRY

SERVES 1

5 fresh or frozen strawberries
⅛ teaspoon spirulina powder

Place all the ingredients in a high-speed blender or NutriBullet with 100ml (3½fl oz/scant ½ cup) water and blend for at least 1 minute. Sieve the elixir through a fine sieve over a jug, then serve in a small glass.

BLACKBERRY, GINGER & ALOE VERA

SERVES 1

5 fresh or frozen blackberries
½cm (¼in) piece of ginger, peeled
2 tablespoons aloe vera juice

Place all the ingredients in a high-speed blender or NutriBullet with 100ml (3½fl oz/scant ½ cup) water and blend for at least 1 minute. Sieve the elixir through a fine sieve over a jug, then serve in a small glass.

ALOE VERA, LIME & COCONUT

SERVES 1

1 tablespoon aloe vera juice
½ fresh lime, peeled and deseeded
100ml (3½fl oz/scant ½ cup)
   coconut milk or coconut water

Place all the ingredients in a high-speed blender or NutriBullet and blend for at least 1 minute. Sieve the elixir through a fine sieve over a jug, then serve in a small glass.

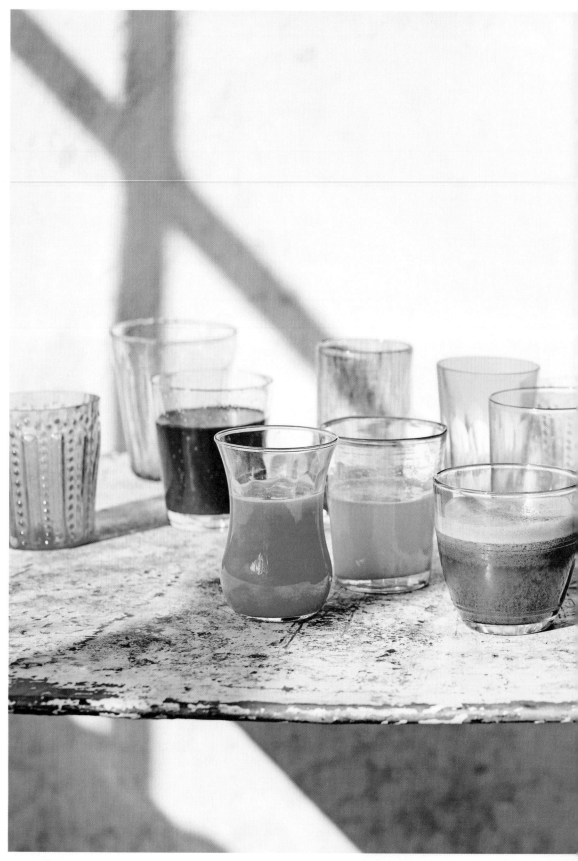

Elixirs pictured in chakra order

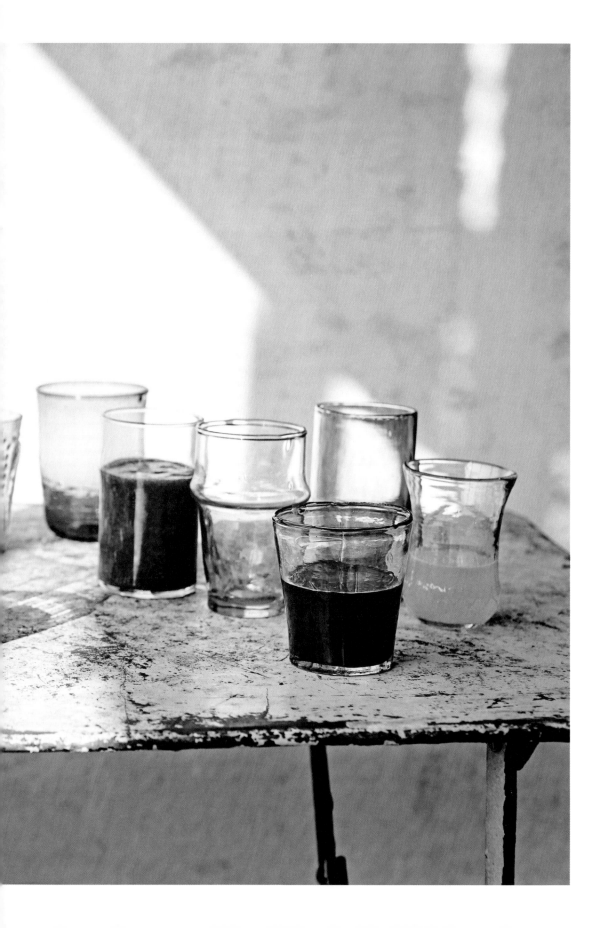

PRE & POST YOGA SNACKS

SMOKED PAPRIKA, CHILLI & LIME CHIA SEED MIXED NUTS (v)

MAKES 2 CUPS

100g (3½oz/scant 1 cup)
   raw cashews
100g (3½oz/¾ cup) raw
   unblanched almonds
100g (3½oz/¾ cup) raw brazil
   nuts, halved
20g (⅔oz/½ cup) coconut flakes
½ teaspoon dried chilli (hot
   pepper) flakes
2 teaspoons smoked paprika
60ml (2fl oz/¼ cup) freshly
   squeezed lime juice
1 tablespoon coconut sugar
1 tablespoon chia seeds
2 teaspoons sea salt
1 teaspoon finely grated lime zest

Preheat oven to 160°C/315°F/Gas 3 and line a baking sheet with baking paper.

Place all the nuts and coconut flakes into a mixing bowl. Add the chilli flakes, smoked paprika, lime juice, coconut sugar, chia seeds and salt. Toss to combine.

Spread out the flavoured nuts on the prepared baking sheet and roast in the oven for 20 minutes, or until golden. Add the lime zest and toss to combine. Allow to cool before serving.

The nut mixture can be kept in an airtight container for up to 1 week.

SUNFLOWER TAMARI CLUSTERS (v)

6 SERVINGS

275g (9¾oz/2 cups)
   sunflower seeds
50g (1¾oz/scant ⅓ cup)
   chia seeds
1 tablespoon ground flaxseed
3 tablespoons toasted sesame oil
3 tablespoons tamari sauce
freshly squeezed juice of 1 lime

Place all the ingredients into a mixing bowl and stir to completely cover the seeds in the liquid ingredients. Once combined, spread the seeds out onto the prepared baking sheet.

Leave to sit at room temperature for 30 minutes, so that the chia seeds can absorb the tamari and sesame oil.

Preheat oven to 180°C/350°F/Gas 4. Line a large baking sheet with baking paper.

Bake in the preheated oven for 20–25 minutes, or until the seeds have turned a golden brown colour and all the liquid has gone from the baking sheet. Remove from the oven and let the seeds cool on the sheet before breaking up in your hands into bite-size clusters and storing in a glass jar or airtight container.

TOASTED SESAME KALE CHIPS (v)

4 SERVINGS

350g (12oz) curly kale, stalks removed and leaves roughly torn
2 tablespoons sesame oil
2 teaspoons tamari sauce
2 teaspoons sesame seeds

Preheat the oven to 200°C/400°F/Gas 6.

Place the kale, sesame oil, tamari and sesame seeds into a large mixing bowl. Toss to coat, then spread out evenly in a single layer over a baking sheet.

Bake in the preheated oven for 6 minutes, or until crisp. Remove from the oven and allow to cool completely on the baking sheet.

GINGERNUT COOKIES (v)

MAKES 6 COOKIES

200g (7oz/2 cups) ground almonds
60g (2oz/¼ cup) coconut sugar
1 tablespoon ground ginger
½ teaspoon ground allspice
a pinch of sea salt
120ml (4fl oz/½ cup) liquid from a can of chickpeas (garbanzo beans)
¼ teaspoon cream of tartar
2 tablespoons maple syrup

Preheat oven to 160°C/315°F/Gas 2–3. Line a baking sheet with baking paper and set aside.

In a large mixing bowl add the ground almonds, coconut sugar, ginger, allspice and salt, stir to combine, then set this aside while you concentrate on the aquafaba.

In a large mixing bowl, put the chickpea liquid (known as aquafaba) and the cream of tartar. Using an electric whisk, beat the liquid until light and fluffy – this should take 3–5 minutes. Stop beating at the point stiff peaks are almost reached. Now add the maple syrup and beat again until stiff peaks form.

Fold half of the aquafaba mixture into the dry mix using a gentle figure of eight motion with your spatula or wooden spoon. Try to combine all the dry ingredients into the aquafaba, then add the rest of the aquafaba and lightly fold again, being careful not to over mix. The mixture should be light and fluffy to touch. If over mixed, the cookies will be dense and overly chewy.

Using an ice cream scoop or large dessertspoon, scoop the mixture onto the prepared baking sheet to make 6 mounds, leaving a 3cm (1¼in) space between each cookie as they will spread slightly.

Bake in the preheated oven for 45 minutes, or until golden and crisp. Remove from the oven and allow to cool completely before touching. Store the cookies in an airtight container to maintain their crisp texture.

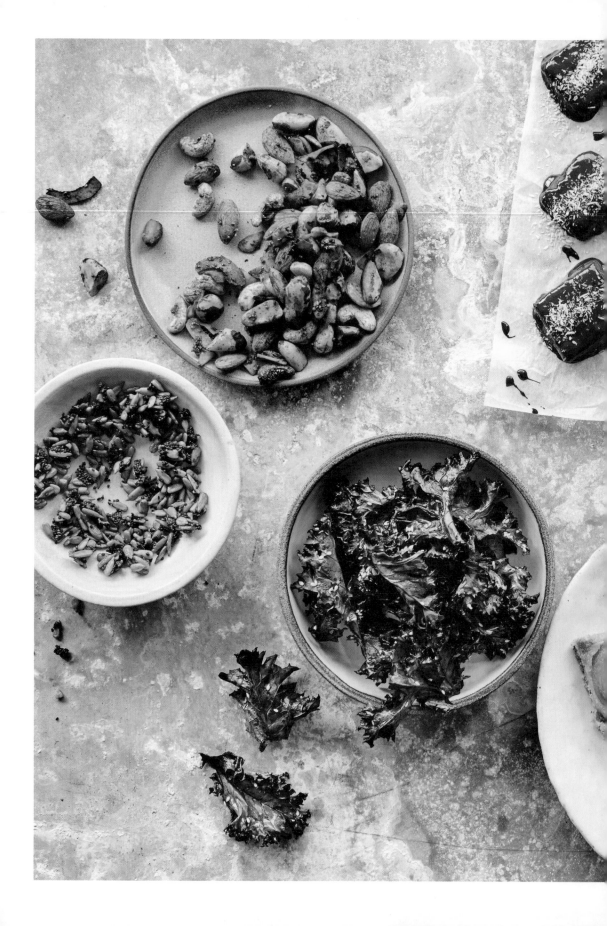

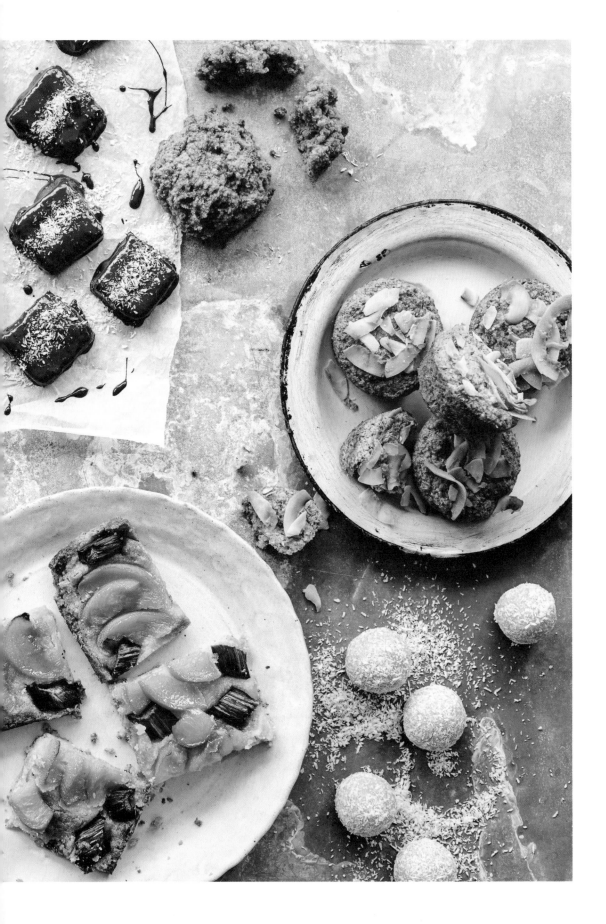

PEACH & RHUBARB ALMOND SQUARES

SERVES 2–4

FOR THE CRUST

100g (3½oz/1 cup) ground
  almonds
3 tablespoons rice flour
2 tablespoons golden caster sugar
  or coconut sugar
2 tablespoons ground flaxseed
⅛ teaspoon salt
50g (1¾oz/3½ tablespoons)
  butter, melted

FOR THE TOPPING

110g (3¾oz/¾ cup) ground
  almonds
1¾ tbsp rice flour
¼ teaspoon salt
65g (2¼oz/⅓ cup) golden caster
  sugar or coconut sugar
80g (2¾oz/5½ tablespoons)
  butter, melted
1 teaspoon vanilla extract
250g (9oz) canned sliced
  peaches in juice, drained
100g (3½oz) rhubarb, chopped
  into 2cm (¾in) lengths

Preheat the oven to 180°C/350°C/Gas 4 and line a 20 x 20cm
(8 x 8in) square baking pan with a sheet of baking paper.

In a mixing bowl, stir together the almond flour, rice flour, sugar,
flaxseed, salt and melted butter until fully combined and there's
no dry ingredients remaining. Press the crust mixture firmly into
the base of the prepared baking pan. Place the baking pan in
the fridge while you prepare the topping.

In a mixing bowl, stir together the ground almonds, rice flour,
salt, sugar, melted butter and vanilla until fully combined. Spread
the topping mixture evenly over the almond base, then press the
peach and rhubarb slices into the topping mixture.

Bake in the preheated oven for 50 minutes, or until golden on
top. Allow to cool completely before cutting into 9 squares.

CHOCOLATE & COCONUT BITES

MAKES 12

180g (6¼oz/2¼ cups) desiccated
  (dried shredded) coconut
60g (2oz/¼ cup) coconut oil,
  melted
2½ tablespoons maple syrup
¼ teaspoon vanilla extract
a pinch of sea salt
100g (3½) dark chocolate, roughly
  chopped

Line a small baking pan or loaf pan with baking paper.

In a mixing bowl, add the desiccated coconut, coconut oil,
maple syrup, vanilla extract and sea salt. Stir to completely coat
all the ingredients. Press this mixture into your baking pan or loaf
pan, making sure it is as firmly packed down as possible. Freeze
for 10 minutes while you melt the chocolate.

Put the chocolate in a heatproof glass bowl. Place the bowl over
a saucepan of simmering water and stir until the chocolate is
melted. Remove the saucepan from the heat.

Remove the coconut from the freezer and cut into 2.5 x 2.5cm
(1 x 1in) squares. Line a baking sheet or plate with baking
paper. Dip the squares into the melted chocolate and place on
the paper. Dip the remaining squares, then refrigerate the bites
until set. Store in the fridge or in a cool environment.

PASSION FRUIT & COCONUT TROPICANA MUFFINS (v)

MAKES 8

70g (2½oz/⅓ cup) coconut oil, melted, plus extra for greasing
2 tablespoons ground flaxseed
120ml (4fl oz/½ cup) maple syrup
230g (8oz/1 cup) peeled and mashed banana (about 2 large bananas)
pulp of 2 passion fruits
1 teaspoon freshly squeezed lemon juice
2 teaspoons baking powder
1 teaspoon bicarbonate of soda (baking soda)
1 teaspoon vanilla extract
½ teaspoon sea salt
90g (3¼oz/¾ cup) spelt flour
80g (2¾oz/¾ cup) ground almonds
70g (2½oz/¾ cup) desiccated (dried shredded) coconut
coconut flakes, to top

Preheat the oven to 160°C/315°F/Gas 2–3 and grease 8 holes of a muffin tray with a thin layer of coconut oil.

In a small mixing bowl, combine the ground flaxseed with 60ml (2fl oz/¼ cup) water. Stir and set aside.

In a large mixing bowl, beat together the melted coconut oil and maple syrup until combined. Add the flaxseed mixture, mashed banana, passion-fruit pulp and lemon juice. Stir to combine using a wooden spoon, making sure to leave a few lumps of banana.

Whisk through the baking powder, bicarbonate of soda, vanilla and salt, then fold in the flour, ground almonds and desiccated coconut and stir to combine.

Divide the batter evenly between the muffin moulds, top with some coconut flakes and bake in the preheated oven for 30 minutes, or until an inserted skewer comes out clean. Once baked, remove the muffins from the oven and allow to cool.

These muffins can be stored in the fridge for up to 1 week, or place in the freezer and defrost whenever you need a little sweet post-yoga snack.

APRICOT, LEMON & CARDAMOM BALLS (v)

MAKES ABOUT 30

350g (12oz/2⅓ cups) dried apricots
150g (5½oz/2 cups) desiccated (dried shredded) coconut, plus a little extra for coating
120g (4¼oz/½ cup) mango purée
½ teaspoon sea salt
100g (3½oz/heaped ¾ cup) raw cashews
¼ teaspoon ground cardamom
freshly grated zest of 1 lemon
3 tablespoons coconut oil

Place all the ingredients in a food processor and process until a smooth, dough-like consistency is reached. The apricots should completely break down and the ingredients will form a ball within the food processor. This can take 5 minutes or more.

Remove the ball from the food processor. Break off small amounts and roll between your palms into balls. Roll each ball in a little desiccated coconut, then refrigerate for 2 hours to cool and set. Store in an airtight container for up to 2 months.

INDEX

Publishing Director: Sarah Lavelle
Commissioning Editor: Céline Hughes
Design and Art Direction: Gemma Hayden
Photographer: Laura Edwards
Food Stylist: Frankie Unsworth
Prop Stylist: Polly Webb-Wilson
Food Stylist Assistants: Sian Williams and Izy Hossack
Cover Lettering: Arielle Gamble
Production Controller: Sinead Hering
Production Director: Vincent Smith

Published in 2019 by Quadrille,
an imprint of Hardie Grant Publishing

Quadrille
52–54 Southwark Street
London SE1 1UN
quadrille.com

Cataloguing in Publication Data: a catalogue record
for this book is available from the British Library.

Text © Kimberly Parsons 2019
Photography © Laura Edwards 2019
Design and layout © Quadrille Publishing Limited 2019

ISBN: 978 1 78713 321 1

Printed in China

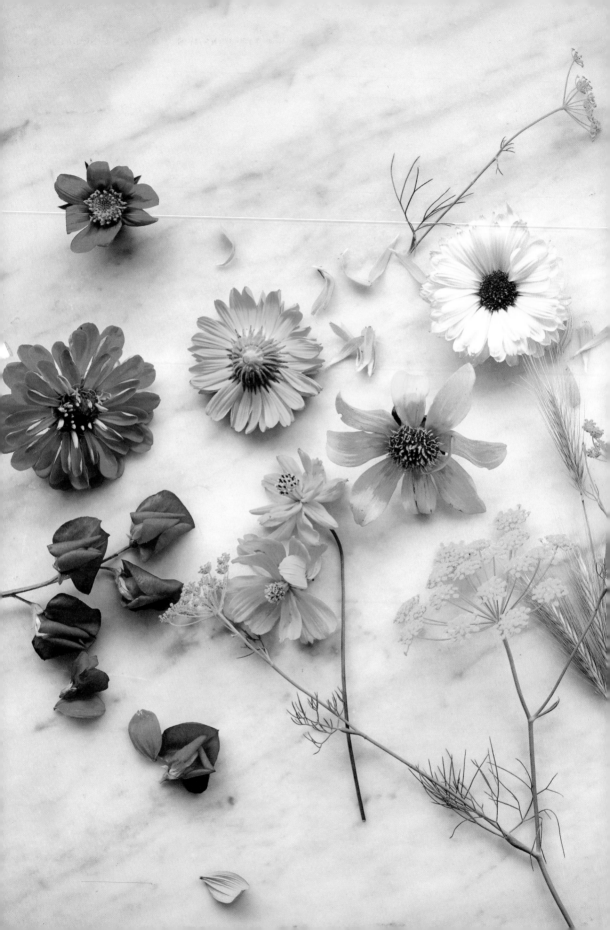

ACKNOWLEDGEMENTS

To Lizaan Joubert: you are the best example of a human being I have had the pleasure of meeting in this lifetime and it is without hesitation that I dedicate this book to you. Not only are you fierce beyond all measure, you are also the most whole-hearted, honest, real and raw woman I know. You have taught me more about myself than 34 birthdays have managed to so far. Thank you for allowing me to be your student in life and sharing your wisdom with me. Our prosecco lunches are some of my fondest memories and I hope we have many more to come.

To Heather Holden-Brown, my agent, and assistant extraordinaire Cara Armstrong: thank you for everything you do for me. Your unwavering belief in and support of my ideas are a constant source of gratitude for me. Without the both of you, I would not be able to do what I love to do.

To Céline, my editor: thank you for seeing what I saw in this book and enabling it to become something I am truly proud of. Your gentle yet thorough skill as an editor gave me the confidence to continue to create, all the while knowing you were guiding this ship with your refined knowledge of how this book needed to reach its target audience.

To Gemma: thank you for your ability to listen to and see my vision for this book. Your beauty as a person, inside and out, is undoubtedly why you are able to produce such beautiful books. Thank you for all the lovely moments we shared on the photo shoot.

To Margaux Durigon, Rebecca Smedley and everyone at Quadrille who has had a part to play in creating this book: I thank you and want to reiterate just how much I love being a part of your family and being one of the lucky authors who get to work with you all.

To Laura Edwards: I have no doubt you were put on this Earth to hold a camera and capture the essence of food. What a privilege it was to work with you and watch your mastery at play. Thank you for making it look effortless and bringing such joy to each day.

Thanks also go to Sam Harris, Laura's photography assistant, and Polly Webb-Wilson, prop stylist, for the gorgeous crystals, wild flowers and overall understanding and enthusiasm for this book.

To Frankie Unsworth, food stylist and wonder-woman with food: I am truly in awe of your knowledge and abilities with food. Thank you for coping with an author who felt very uncomfortable outside of the kitchen for the shoot. You made every plate look more delicious than I could ever have hoped. I feel truly lucky to have had you on our team. Thank you also to Sian Williams and Izy Hossack for all your help in the kitchen on those incredibly hot shoot days and for troubleshooting when the recipes where not playing ball with us.

To Georgie Day: thank you for all the ridiculous shopping trips to supermarkets in foreign countries. For our endless conversations about food and for being my sounding board, diligent recipe tester and best kitchen assistant ever. Your exuberant energy fills every kitchen we find ourselves in with high vibes and great conversation. I am so grateful to have found you and look forward to seeing your growth and where our adventures take us next.

To Tom: thank you for being my courage and belief when I couldn't find my own. For being the man that you are, every day without faltering, for writing the chapters of life with me and giving me everything I have ever wanted and more.

And to all of you guys: this book is for you! Without your support and enthusiasm for *The Yoga Kitchen*, I wouldn't be here today. Thank you for all your comments and excitement over the last few years. I feel honoured that you allow me into your kitchens with these recipes and I wish you all good health and calmer living as you go forth and journey through this life. Thank you for allowing me to be a part of it x

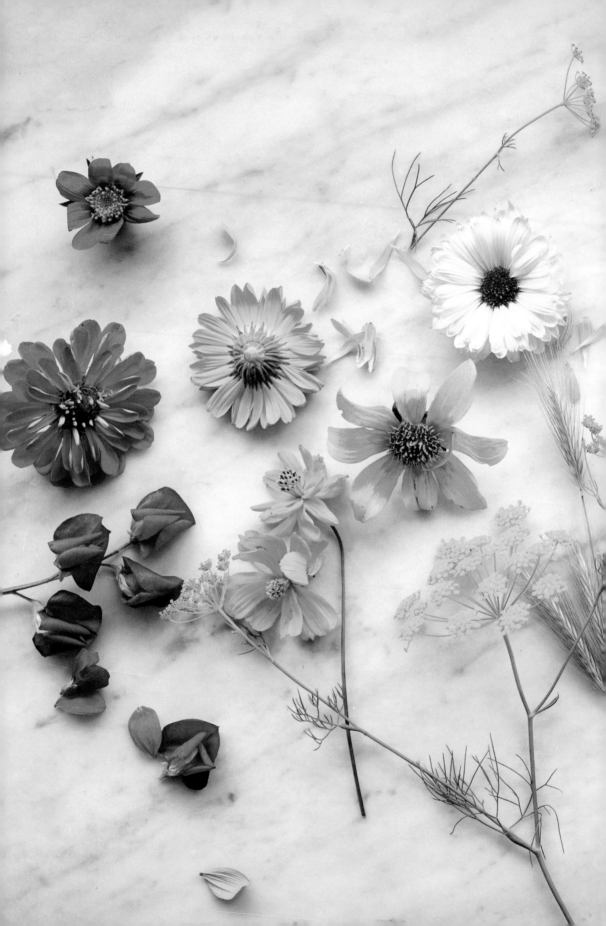